Off My Chest

Off My Chest

A Breast Cancer Memoir of Hellfire, Healing, and Radical Acceptance

Jill Wilson

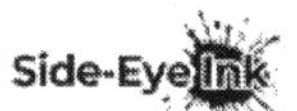

Published by Side-Eye Ink
Longmont, Colorado

This memoir reflects the author's personal experiences. It is not intended to provide medical, psychological, or therapeutic advice. Readers should consult qualified professionals regarding their own health, mental health, or treatment decisions.

This is a work of nonfiction. Some names and identifying details have been changed to protect privacy. The experiences, reflections, and opinions expressed in this book are the author's own.

Cover design: Jill Wilson
Author photo: Jakob Vuolo

Publisher's Cataloging-in-Publication Data
(Provided by Cassidy Cataloguing Services, Inc.).
Names: Wilson, Jill, author.

Title: Off my chest : a breast cancer memoir of hellfire, healing, and radical acceptance / Jill Wilson.

Description: First edition. | [Longmont, Colorado] : Side-Eye Ink, [2026]

Identifiers: ISBN: 9798994285008 (paperback) | 9798994285022 (hardcover) | 9798994285015 (eBook)

Subjects: LCSH: Wilson, Jill. | Breast--Cancer--Patients--Biography. | Breast--Cancer--Patients--Psychological aspects. | Breast--Cancer--Treatment. | Medical care--United States. | Breast cancer patients' writings. | LCGFT: Autobiographies. | BISAC: BIOGRAPHY & AUTOBIOGRAPHY / Memoirs. | HEALTH & FITNESS / Diseases / Cancer.

Classification: LCC: RC280.B8 W55 2026 | DDC: 616.994490092--dc23

Printed in the United States of America

First edition, 2025

For Scott—
my constant in chaos and calm.

"This isn't a comeback story. It's a story of becoming."

Table of Contents

Author's Note

This book is about disruption—of the body, the system, and every tidy narrative I was supposed to follow after cancer. It spans multiple diagnoses and the long middle that came after them, moving between the before, the during, and the aftermath in a way that mirrors how I actually lived it: nonlinear, looping, sometimes chaotic, sometimes unexpectedly tender. I wrote it as honestly as I could, with all the humor, dark wit, ambivalence, and identity-based rebellion that helped me survive.

These pages blend personal experience with systemic critique, because cancer doesn't happen in a vacuum. It happens inside a healthcare system built to exhaust us, inside cultural myths that demand bravery at all costs, inside families and relationships that bend and strain under the weight of fear. I'm a human rights advocate as well as a patient, so you'll feel that perspective here too: curiosity toward the self, compassion for others, and a steady refusal to look away from the structural forces shaping our private lives.

Some of the people in this book are composites, and certain details, timelines, and conversations have been altered to protect privacy—my own and everyone else's. These events are described to the best of my recollection, which means memory does some of the storytelling with me. Trauma has a way of rearranging time, so I've let the narrative follow truth instead of chronology.

This book isn't a medical guide, a treatment plan, or a roadmap for anyone else's healing. Survivorship is not uniform, linear, or neatly resolved, and I won't pretend it is here. Please seek professional medical or mental-health support for your own care. My story is mine, not a universal template and not a prescription.

What I hope you'll find in these pages is connection: the kind that comes from telling the truth without making it pretty. If you've lived through illness, trauma, uncertainty, or the aftermath where everyone else moves on—you're not alone. This is a story about the messy work of staying human when life refuses to go back to normal, and about choosing, again and again, to rewrite what survival can mean.

PART I

When Ordinary Life Fell Out of Orbit

Pink Smocks & Galaxies

The Galaxy in My Breast

I wasn't going to get bad news in a stupid pink smock. Those things are designed to strip you—literally and figuratively—of power. You stop being a person and become a procedure. A statistic. A barcode wrapped in pastel. I pulled my T-shirt back on, reclaiming the smallest slice of dignity. The cotton settled against my skin like armor. I needed to feel like myself—grounded enough to ask questions and outmaneuver fear. That T-shirt gave me a sliver of stability in a world that was already shifting.

That's my tell: when the ground drops, I reach for agency and language.

I'd just finished a diagnostic mammogram—painstakingly precise from every conceivable angle my boob could be flattened. Now I sat alone in a dim consultation room waiting for the radiologist. The air felt cold. I already knew something was wrong. The technicians had been too quiet, too careful. No jokes about awkward poses, no apologizing for the panini-press level of boob compression. The vibes were all wrong, and my body knew it.

The radiologist entered, calm but serious, eyes connecting with mine. He dimmed the room further until the glow of two monitors provided most of the light. With a few quick keystrokes, my breast appeared in duplicate—an X-ray constellation. He pointed to last year's mammogram first, identifying a few unremarkable dots. Then he moved to the new one, tracing a full arc of brightness across the screen with his finger.

"See this?" he said. "It's… unusual."

Hundreds of tiny lights glittered across my breast, no solid mass, just a sprawling galaxy. He circled each end of the arc and admitted he couldn't tell where it began or ended. The image was breathtaking. Impossible. Unnatural in the way supernovas probably are right before they collapse.

He mentioned a same-day biopsy. I glanced at the clock—2:30 p.m., Tuesday. I was supposed to start my hospital shift in thirty minutes. And tomorrow? Out of the question. We were leaving for Mexico in three days. I needed to dive. To sail. To make memories with my family. My brain started negotiating like it was a hostage. My body needed to hold it together just a little longer.

On the outside, I nodded politely. On the inside: Seriously? I'm on the clock in twenty-five minutes. My Outlook calendar does not include "malignancy" this week.

I scheduled the biopsy for two weeks later, two days after we'd return. If I was about to enter a new reality called Cancer, I was damn sure going to live one last perfect week in this one.

I didn't know it yet, but survivorship would become a long negotiation with language—what people called me, what they expected, what I refused.

Cosmic Jalapeños

In the two weeks between the mammogram and the biopsy, my husband, Scott, and I took our kids to Akumal. It was the kind of trip you hope burns into everyone's long-term memory—the smells of salt and mango, the wet slap of snorkel fins, the kind of connection you can only get when you're all in the same water, the same sun, the same time. We dove with cuttlefish under a blanket of bioluminescence. Freedived in sacred cenotes, sunlight piercing the surface in holy beams. Kayaked through ancient mangroves where everything felt older than time itself.

The highlight? Swimming with three whale sharks. I paddled so hard my lungs threatened mutiny, but in that moment—surging beside those gentle giants—I felt like I was flying. Otherworldly. Magical. Alive.

Each evening, we gathered for long, lingering dinners that stretched past sunset. We'd all order something different and share everything. Usually, one of every dessert on the menu made it to the table—flan, key lime pie, spicy chocolate cake, cinnamon-dusted sopaipillas, tres leches. One fork at a time, we'd pass each plate clockwise, savoring a bite, ranking favorites like dessert critics who took the job very seriously. The table filled with laughter, coconut, and mayhem—our own small ritual of joy. Exploring food together became its own adventure, and the conversations were priceless.

I was collecting beauty like it could inoculate me.

Still, joy and dread shared the same reef. Beneath the awe, anxiety pressed from the edges like a current. Even as I swam, I knew what was waiting at home. I just refused to let it claim this week. It was the kids' first trip abroad. I wanted them to have one album of memory where I wasn't a diagnosis in the foreground. I wanted to be their mom, not their impending patient. I needed our inside jokes to survive the months ahead. I needed their laughter to have a "before."

I thought about that tension constantly—how beauty and fear can coexist, how the body can hold both simultaneously. I recalled a previous dive trip with my son, Max, when we planted coral for reef restoration. The current was just strong enough that each of us had to cling to the reef with one hand while planting baby corals with the other. At one point, I reached behind me to grab another coral from the bucket, but instead of prickly texture, I felt something smooth—soft, almost velvety.

I turned my head. My fingers were resting on the nose of a curious nurse shark.

Time slowed. Panic pulsed, then receded. I couldn't scream or thrash—I had a regulator in my mouth. I went limp, surrendered to the current, my fingers still tethered to the reef. The shark hovered, watching, unbothered, a tight-lipped judge of our clumsy human intrusion. For five long minutes it stayed, shifting slightly for a better angle. The filtered light danced across its back, creating a mosaic of movement—each reflection gone before I could memorize it.

Fear, awe, surrender—all in one breath. A preview, though I didn't know it then, of what was coming.

Home smelled like laundry and looming.

The day before my biopsy, I took the kids to a Colorado Rockies game. Late summer, hot enough to melt reason. Sunscreen, lemonade, the smell of hoppy beer and popcorn oil. The guys behind us were hilarious, loud, instantly magnetic—queer, friendly, celebrating a birthday. Before long, we were a collective, cheering and sweating together.

"What do you do?" one of them asked.

"I work at a hospital," I said.

He grinned. "Same. I'm a breast surgeon."

"Oh," I said, pretending this was casual information. "That must be hard, dealing with cancer every day."

"When we catch it early," he said, "outcomes are really good." I stared at him. There are 47,000 seats in Coors Field. I could have sat next to a plumber, a CPA, a mascot—anyone. But the universe, in its infinite sense of humor, had seated me directly in front of a breast surgeon.

Then he turned back to his nachos like he hadn't just delivered a cosmic telegram in jalapeño cheese.

"Early would have been last season," I muttered into my lemonade.

Core Samples & Controlled Burns

The next morning, I showed up for my biopsy. I'd had two in the few years before—both false alarms. But this time, the nurse handed me two pamphlets: one outlining the procedure, and another featuring a woman in a headscarf holding a mug like it contained federal secrets. The title: Your Journey Through Breast Cancer.

I handed that one back. "Hard pass. We don't even know if I have cancer yet."

That was optimism talking. Or denial. A fine, blurry line.

Inside the biopsy room, the air smelled faintly of antiseptic and printer toner. The table beside me was the problematic kind—the one with the cutouts so your breasts can dangle through like awkward sacrifices. The tech tucked a warmed blanket around my shoulders—an unearned mercy. The radiologist narrated as she worked, like competence could soften the whole thing: "You'll hear a loud click. That's the core. Pressure, not pain." The machine buzzed; the monitor threw blue light onto the floor.

I stayed stoic but funny—my default setting under pressure. The team offered quiet compassion, space to cry, or distraction. I went for distraction. Jokes. Questions. A full TED Talk on efficiency mid-procedure.

About halfway through, as the core needle suctioned tissue, I noticed a tiny inefficiency. They were prepping to clear the tray and reset for the second tumor site.

"Why break the sterile field?" I asked, eyeballing the tray and trying not to move. "If you drop the second packet of gauze on the corner now, you can pivot to the second site without re-gloving."

The radiologist paused, looked at the tray, and laughed.

"You'd be a great fit for our team," she said.

"Perfect," I replied. "Do employees get a discount on pathology reports?"

The radiology team laughed, and somehow that laughter made the room bearable. Humor was my anesthesia. If I could manage the room, the room couldn't manage me. (My idea worked, by the way. Gold star.)

They placed the marker clips, applied pressure, then a bandage that looked wildly underqualified for the job was wrapped around me. The tech explained aftercare. "Ice twenty minutes on, twenty minutes off. No heavy lifting."

"Define heavy," I said. "Existential dread? Grabbing groceries?"

"Just the groceries," she deadpanned, and I decided I loved her.

The Call, the Collapse, the Nasal Strip

Four days later, the call came.

My longtime physician assistant—someone I trusted completely—was on the line. Her voice was tentative and kind, the way people sound when they're holding your parachute. She gave me the news. I asked for the pathology report and she sent it through the patient portal. I opened it, scanning for the word I already knew was there.

There it was: carcinoma. Then: multifocal. Grade 3.

I lasted maybe five minutes before my voice cracked and the floodgates opened. She spoke softly about next steps, that an oncology nurse would be in touch soon, but I barely heard her. My mouth went dry like I'd swallowed sand. I was trying to breathe. And I kept thinking, What the fuck is multifocal?

Scott was on a work trip in Alabama. I called twice—no answer. Finally, I texted: Call me when you can.

When he called a short time later, I didn't ease in. "I have breast cancer," I blurted, then started crying. How are you supposed to share this news? How are you supposed to receive it? He gave space for the moment and listened. We stayed on the line together, me sniffling, him struggling to stay composed. Until words felt possible again. Then he booked the next flight home.

That night we sat on the couch, holding each other in heavy silence. My face was so swollen from crying that I had to sleep propped up, breathing through a nasal strip like a melodramatic raccoon. My body felt weighted, hollowed, impossible.

From my pillow fortress, I stared at my charcoal gray scrubs draped over the bedroom chair. My hospital ID badge was still clipped to the collar, sporting two gold star stickers—a grim souvenir from the biopsy team for being a "good patient." I looked at them and felt a hot spike of grief. I was nine months away from finishing my respiratory therapy program. I had left a two-decade career in financial services to wear those scrubs. I had traded spreadsheets for breath—and now breath was the thing I couldn't trust. I was supposed to be the one walking into trauma rooms to help people breathe, not the one propped up struggling to catch her own breath.

On the nightstand, a framed selfie watched over us. Scott and I, windblown on a hiking trail near Santa Fe, fueled by food truck tacos because every restaurant had been closed. We had married in March 2020, right as the world shut down for COVID. Our marriage had been forged in that global chaos—a private joy while the world fell apart.

Our kids were thriving—college, high school, middle school—all of them coming into themselves. We were busy, happy, exhausted in the best possible way. The kind of ordinary fullness you don't realize is extraordinary until it's threatened.

I looked from the photo to the scrubs to the dark window. I didn't want to leave this life. I wanted to stay.

But the galaxy inside me had begun to pulse with its own light, dazzling and dangerous.

A galaxy burned in my breast; resistance bloomed everywhere else.

Diagnosis Delivered

By morning, resistance put on reading glasses. If I couldn't control the threat, I could at least learn its grammar.

Crash Course in Cancer

Cancer didn't ease me in. One day I was looking up dive footage on YouTube and planning my hospital shifts. The next, I was decoding pathology like my life depended on it. Because it did.

No one warned me I'd need to become fluent in a new language overnight: Ki-67, comedonecrosis, multifocal, microinvasive, grade 3, tumor board. It wasn't survival prep; it was a pop quiz in a tongue I didn't speak. I googled each term, made a ruthless list for the oncology nurse, and fell down rabbit holes where the footnotes were longer than the studies. Microinvasive ductal carcinoma—uncommon enough to make the tumor board lean in.

My questions came fierce and fast. What exactly is happening in my breast? What are the odds? Lumpectomy or mastectomy—and if mastectomy, one side or both? Will I need radiation? Endocrine therapy? ER/PR statuses? Will treatment slam me into early menopause and poke the hornet's nest of my autoimmune disease? Every answer opened three new possibilities. It kept my brain busy while my heart tried not to implode.

Learning the language was one thing. Living inside it came with forms.

Stationery for the Apocalypse

The oncology nurse was kind and composed. She answered a handful of my forty-seven questions and tried—more than once—to ask how I was doing. I didn't have an answer for that yet, so I clung to logistics. A tiny slice of control. She scheduled an MRI for the next day to map extent and look at lymph nodes. I didn't cry on the phone with her. Maybe because I'd emptied the tank the day before. Maybe because she did this every day and carried a calm I could borrow for five minutes.

At the imaging center, I filled out the same medical questionnaire I'd filled out a hundred times before. But this time my pen paused, and my eyes flooded. Have you ever received a cancer diagnosis? I checked the box. I turned to Scott. "Well, it's official. I'm a statistic."

Next came the MRI—fifty-five minutes of immobility while magnets sliced my body into data. The table ridge dug under my ribs; the vibrations rattled my brain. Despite the high-tech everything, the noise-canceling headphones were so shitty I couldn't tell if the playlist was jazz, techno, or a Gregorian chant remixed by a Roomba. The machine banged and chirped and thrummed. I counted my breaths like a metronome: four in, six out.

When it ended, the tech handed me a giant binder. "It's your box," she said brightly. A pink cancer box. Inside: tabs for every appointment, result, medication, and medical professional. Outside: black script announcing BREAST CANCER to the world. Another staffer chimed in, "Is your husband taking you to dinner? You deserve it!" She recommended a fancy steakhouse next door. Because nothing pairs with a new diagnosis quite like overpriced surf and turf.

We got burgers. I cried into mine. Nobody stared. The cheeseburger crowd understands grief.

By the time we got home, the binder felt like it was shouting at me. I tossed the cancer box into the trash with the greasy fry wrapper—they belonged together. It was either that or duct-tape the binder in brown paper and label it: DEFINITELY NOT CANCER, JUST A BINDER OF JOY, which felt a little too Pinterest for the occasion.

Now, there was nothing to do but wait. The room finally got still enough for feeling.

Hold Music & Rage

The next morning the MRI report posted: axillary nodes "prominent." Translation: enlarged, possibly involved. I needed an ultrasound. A breast surgeon. An oncologist. A plan. And in the meantime, I got hold music.

I made cancer a full-time job. I buried myself in research, printed studies, annotated margins. I showed up to every appointment with my black notebook—doctors' names and roles, question lists, answers, protocols, side effects, locations, call times. Gaining knowledge made me feel in control—

especially while everything else spun. Logistics was armor. If I just managed it hard enough, maybe I wouldn't have to feel it.

The feelings rolled in anyway.

On Day Four, the adrenaline wore off. The appointment flurry quieted. The inbox slowed. My logistical armor clattered to the floor, and the weight landed where it always does: on the body.

I got pissed. I was supposed to be starting my final year of respiratory therapy school, not googling survival curves and dose-dense regimens. I grieved my timeline, my plans, my illusion that I was in control. Some moments I felt it in my gut: I've got this. Seconds later: How the hell am I going to get through this?

I cried because I cared about losing my hair—and then felt ashamed for caring about something so "vain" when my life was at stake. It turns out vanity doesn't evaporate just because your life is on fire.

I wondered what my body would look like. Would I recognize myself? Love myself? Accept myself?

When You Can't Do It All

Telling people was its own kind of hell. My kids. My stepkids. Our parents. Each conversation carried two jobs: inform and console. I said the words, "I have cancer," and watched faces droop. Then I tried to hold them up while I was falling apart.

Friends. Co-workers. Extended family. Their heartbreak became mine. The emotional toll compounded until I felt hollowed out—like I was donating parts of myself one conversation at a time.

And while I was busy managing everyone else's grief, my life kept asking for output—deadlines, schedules, competency—as if cancer was an inconvenience I could politely resolve.

The fall semester started five days after my biopsy. I got the confirmation call on day three of school—before surgery, before an oncologist, before I even knew what "Stage 1" would cost.

It was supposed to be my final year in a demanding respiratory therapy program I loved. I was juggling school and shifts at a Level 1 trauma center where I thrived caring for patients. Then my calendar turned medical: scans, labs, surgeons. The math stopped working. Healing and education were on a collision course.

I told myself I could do it all. I'd done hard things before. But school was already intense on my best days. How was I going to scrub in for clinicals with drains under my shirt? I knew just enough about medicine to be dangerous—and very, very afraid.

I met with my program director in the first week—the fourth day, I think. I planned to be composed. Instead, I cried. Then I wiped my face and told her the truth. She asked questions I couldn't yet answer and then said the words I didn't know I needed: "We'll get you through—clinicals, licensure, the whole finish line." I nodded, grateful and grieving in the same breath.

But that night in the kitchen, I told Scott I needed to pause school. My chest tightened like a fist and also loosened, just a little. I could feel both things at once: the ache and the resolve. It felt like watching a whole year of plans blur on the calendar, the ink bleeding into one gray smear, while my own hand held the pen that drew a hard line through the semester.

Surgery was coming. Recovery would be real. Clinicals—hands-on, physical, relentless—would be out of the question. We didn't even know about chemo yet. Still, the decision was clear.

I emailed my professors and classmates. Responses poured in—kindness, prayers, offers to share notes. People told me I'd made a difference. It was gutting and humbling and not at all the ceremony I imagined at the end of a degree. Part of me wanted to disappear into a burrito blanket and be no one's inspiration. Part of me was deeply relieved to have named a limit.

I wouldn't graduate with my cohort. That stung. I thought I was signing up for a four-month detour: diagnosed in August, recovered by December. But when the tears cleared, I spotted a different route: enroll in a late-start online class at Metro State toward my lifestyle medicine degree, continue through the spring semester. I'd pick up respiratory therapy next fall. My timeline moved. My feet didn't.

At that point, 'early' still sounded like a rescue. I didn't understand the fine print yet. There's nothing simple about breast cancer.

This too, I learned, is cancer.

A Body Made of Buckshot

One week after diagnosis, Scott and I met the breast surgeon. Smart, kind, zero fluff—my people. She walked through the biopsy report, line by line.

My cancer had been busy breaking rules: it had nibbled beyond the milk duct, fast-talked hormones, and replicated like it was on commission. Ki-67—the speedometer for cell division—over 30% is high. Mine was 89%. Eighty-nine.

The "galaxy" of dots on my mammogram wasn't just stellar; it was pathology—a scatter of microtumors across the breast. No lumpectomy. No "just take the lump and go." The plan: bilateral, nipple-sparing mastectomy with immediate direct-to-implant reconstruction. I'd suspected as much. It offered the best odds of clearing disease. Low enough that she said "1–2%" local recurrence risk out loud.

Hearing it out loud still sent a tremor through me. I forced a smile and nodded while Scott took notes. The voice in my gut whispered, This is real. Your body will never be the same.

After a minute of texting, my surgeon returned to the conversation. "Surgery in nine days."

A couple hours later, we met the plastic surgeon on the other side of that text. The office looked like a spa inside a fashion magazine—bright, serene, everyone glowing like they'd been lit from within. Our consult opened with a personalized slide: WELCOME, JILL WILSON. It felt bizarre and comforting. It was a whirlwind. Photos. Measurements. Vitals. History. A step-by-step walkthrough of the operation. Every question answered without condescension. The plan: one operation, one recovery, faster path to endocrine therapy. Bonus: I wouldn't have to see myself without breasts.

Acceptance, it turned out, often arrived dressed as logistics.

The Boob Preservation Society

Apprehension about my post-surgery body was loud. I swung between curiosity and dread like a pendulum. Would I feel like a stranger in my own skin? Would I mourn? Would Scott still desire me? Would I desire me? Would I care?

A photographer friend offered to do a sexy farewell shoot so I could "preserve the memory" of my breasts. A keepsake for the boobs that tried to kill me. Hard pass. I wanted them gone, not bronzed. We could burn a candle for these bitches later.

Still, a thought needled: if I skip the goodbye, do I skip the grief? Was I brave, or just world-class at compartmentalizing?

I staged my own farewell: not photos, but a solitude minute with a hand over each breast. A simple inventory. Thank you for hanging around all these years. For sex. For never fitting right in sports bras. For the way you hated underwire. Not a shrine. Just a nod.

Questions or not, the calendar didn't balk. It was time to trade hypotheticals for scalpels.

Do I Still Have Boobs?

Surgery day. The OR lights were star-bright; a metallic tang crept into my mouth. I drifted off. In the part my body remembers but my mind doesn't, the breast surgeon injected dye into my breast to map the sentinel lymph nodes. Three glowed blue and came out, along with 99% of my breast tissue. The surgeons worked in tandem, tag-teaming breast to breast to shorten anesthesia time and trauma.

When I woke, my head was foggy and there was an IV in my neck, irritating and impossible to ignore. Both of my arm veins had blown just before the first scalpel incision, forcing the anesthesiologist to use my left external jugular—after an issue with the right jugular. I looked and felt like a very recent, very unhappy vampire victim. But at least the surgery had happened.

As soon as Scott walked in, I asked him the only question that mattered: "Do I still have boobs?"

I couldn't confirm it. My neck wouldn't bend with the IV line, and when I reached down… nothing. Numbness. He said yes. I needed proof. The nurse explained they'd used a nerve block; feeling would be late to the party. I still needed proof. He offered to unwrap the bandages so Scott could take a picture.

Honestly? Perfect.

The first glimpse of my new chest arrived via Samsung. I stared at the screen. Not the body I'd known. Not a horror show either. Just… different. A future I hadn't met yet.

The photo was a relief. Later that night, however, there was a brief horror-movie cameo. I screamed for Scott from the bathroom. My pee was Smurf-blue. What in the holy hell?! Apparently, sentinel node dye takes the scenic route out of your system. For two full days. I texted at least five people. I told anyone who would listen that I was peeing blue. I stand by that comedy.

With the surgery behind me, the horizon widened from incision to treatment plans.

Ritual & Tide

Recovery became a routine of drains to empty, pillows to reposition, and meds that worked until they didn't. I fashioned a shower lanyard out of will and string. Nothing humbles like clipping plastic drain bulbs to your body and calling it fashion.

In the space between nurses' calls and Netflix autopilot, I stumbled onto Tig Notaro's stand-up—the one where she walks onstage and says it plain: breast cancer. She'd been thriving—new show, momentum—and then, on the heels of a systemic infection and grieving her mom, the plot turned. The way she held joy and devastation simultaneously made me feel seen.

Then she made a joke about the "more than you can handle" cliché that was so wrong and so right I howled.

I watched it five times. Sometimes I laughed until I snorted. Sometimes I cried. It was emotional yoga. Tig didn't peddle inspiration; she was raw and ridiculous and real. Her audacity gave me permission to have my own. Something shifted. I stopped feeling like a victim. Not because I'd conquered anything, but because I recognized myself again. Alive in the shit of life. Maybe this wasn't a tragedy I had to overcome so much as a truth I could live inside. Maybe cancer was part of my story, not the whole damn book.

The Oncologist, the Oracle

I met my oncologist before surgery and liked her immediately.

She entered the room with the kind of confidence that didn't need volume. Assured. Warm face. A quick smile that said, I do hard things for a living and you're safe with me. She made eye contact—actual eye contact, not the drive-by glance at my forehead—and introduced her scribe, explaining why she was there. Not as a shadow, but as a second set of hands so my doctor could keep her eyes on me, not on a keyboard.

Her hair was swept back behind her ear, sometimes caught in a clip like she'd pinned away anything that might get in the way of the work. She spoke in plain language first. She owned the truth without dressing it up: my case was unusual, and applying population data to one very specific body—mine—was a blunt tool. She admitted she was reluctant to share numbers because numbers can masquerade as certainty. Then she asked questions that had nothing to do with tumors and everything to do with me. Who I was in the real world. What I did. What mattered. What I needed to keep intact.

Based on what we knew then, she thought I could likely skip chemo and radiation—five years of endocrine therapy to starve any hormone-hungry stragglers. I exhaled like my lungs had been holding a grudge. We were talking practicalities, not doom. A plan with verbs.

Also—say it—I was relieved at the thought of keeping my hair.

After surgery, I came into the oncology follow-up carrying a small, fragile hope. My oncologist started with a simple question. "Has your breast surgeon reviewed the pathology with you?"

"Yes," I said. "Clean margins. Clear nodes."

She nodded, then looked back at the report in front of her, and her tone shifted—not alarmed, just… precise.

"And the tumors," she said.

Tumors. Plural.

I blinked. "What tumors?"

The room tilted—just a sudden, sick vertigo that made everything feel slightly too far away. How could I be back at spinning so soon? We had to step back. Start from the beginning. Rewind the tape.

That's how I learned about the hidden tumors: two small ones, 3 mm and 10 mm, tucked inside the tissue like secrets. They hadn't shown up on the mammogram, ultrasound, or MRI. My sentinel nodes were clear, yes, and my official staging still landed at 1A because the tumors were small. But the fact that aggressive cells could slip past all that high-tech screening was a gut-punch. It made the cancer feel less like a lump and more like a behavior—ninja-like and busy, moving in the blind spots while everyone applauded the "clean margins" headline.

That's when the plan lost its straight line.

Next came Oncotype testing. One of those modern-medicine marvels I would've found genuinely fascinating if it hadn't been my future on the table. A sample of my tumor tissue went off to a lab to have my specific biology perform on command. My tumor's genetics, my cancer's personality, run through a scoring system—so my entire body didn't have to perform. At least not yet.

It felt like tarot, except the deck was made of chromosomes and the reader wore a lab coat. We pulled cards anyway: Recurrence Risk. Chemo Benefit. The Tower. My life reduced to a score that would decide whether we'd throw everything we had at microscopic stragglers or keep the treatment plan contained to pills and time.

Then waiting. Surgery was "done," but my nervous system didn't get the memo. I tried to heal while my mind stayed on alert, listening for the next sentence that would rearrange my life.

I asked my oncologist for her gut opinion—before the score came back, before the cards were fully dealt.

She held my gaze. "With how aggressive your cells are," she said, "I want us to be prepared for chemo."

Shit.

Heat rushed my face. My lungs stalled. Then breath returned, shaky and insistent, like my body was reminding me it still had a job. The protocol kept shifting. Fine. I'd pivot. The plan wasn't the point.

Outrage kept my knees from buckling long enough to make the next call.

At home there was a new ritual: Scott made coffee I would forget to drink. I held the questions. He held me.

What mattered was the grip—and the fact that I still had one.

Stage 1, But Complicated as Hell

Surprise! It's Chemo

The next appointment with the oncologist felt like finding mold behind a freshly painted wall.

We started with the basics I'd been waiting to hear: ER positive. PR positive. Hormone-hungry. HER2 negative. Treatable, yes—also stubborn.

Then came Oncotype. The score landed hard. Thirty-seven. Aggressive biology with a real appetite for trouble —high enough to make "early stage" sound like a technicality, high enough to put chemo on the table.

I wanted to say, Right. Next step. What I managed was a nod that pretended not to be a flinch.

The fear wasn't abstract. It lived in the immediate now. I was terrified of not pulling my weight—of becoming a mom who couldn't mother, a partner who couldn't partner. Would I get frail? Would I recover? How would I be changed? Would I make it through treatment without becoming someone my family had to carry? I wasn't thinking in five-year curves. I was thinking in dinners, rides, homework, laundry—ordinary life—and whether chemo would take my hands off the steering wheel.

People hear Stage 1 and exhale, like it's the "good kind" of cancer. Stage 1 still makes you a person who plastic-wraps their chest before breakfast.

The Chemo Cocktail

At the next visit we got specific: TC—Taxotere and Cytoxan. Four cycles, three weeks apart. Chemo served in neat intervals, like anyone's body has ever respected a calendar invite.

My oncologist was gentle, clear, and not in the business of euphemisms. She explained why these drugs fit my subtype, then walked me through the side effects: nausea, fatigue, hair loss, mouth sores, nerve pain. There would be a delayed white blood cell booster, Neulasta, to keep me out of the fever danger zone.

"We'll manage as we go," she said, which is medicine for: We'll adjust once your body tells us how mad it is.

We toured the infusion center: serious, sterile, lined with recliners and IV poles, the windows politely framing Pikes Peak. In November that view usually makes you feel small in an existential way. In this room, it just made everything feel colder. Most patients were older—scarves neat, blankets tucked.

I saw myself in the window: tan from summer hikes and river days, hair long and familiar. This couldn't be my room. I was still young. I didn't belong there. My diagnosis was indifferent.

I started to sob. Not polite tears—an ugly, no-face-left collapse. I buried my head in Scott's chest. He cried too. A nurse came over and said, "There's no shame in crying here."

I nodded, but shame was already busy. I felt exposed, like I'd been caught impersonating someone stoic. I was falling apart. I didn't know yet that shedding is part of treatment: hair, eyebrows, illusions.

Chemo Season

Chemo started just before the holidays, because nothing says festive like gingerbread-scented nausea and sprinkles of hair.

A port went into my chest—because my veins are dramatic and chemo is not a negotiation. Hardware helped, but it didn't make chemo gentle.

A chemo day started with lidocaine—if I remembered. I'd smear a blob of it over the port site, cover it with self-sealing plastic wrap like I was prepping leftovers, and pretend this was normal. Scott drove. He brought two backpacks: his real one with the computer, and the chemo bag—packed like we were hiking straight into Taxotere.

Inside: frozen mitts and socks in a lunchbox cooler, frozen grapes for my mouth, a small blanket from a friend, Qwixx and Quiddler, earbuds, my cancer notebook—the essentials.

First stop was vitals and a blood draw. Then a quick check-in with my oncologist or the nurse practitioner: How are you doing? Any questions? Side effects? Then off to the infusion room, where I signed in and chose a recliner like it was the only agency left to me. I always picked the ones with fewer people nearby. In a room with no privacy, this is what I could afford.

I wore my Death Cab for Cutie sweatshirt every time. It kept me warm and made the port accessible. It also felt like a tiny insistence: I'm still me. Even here.

Shoes off. Feet up. Scott unpacked the blanket and the frozen gear like we'd trained for this. We always arrived with a to-do list—Christmas presents, meal planning, and the small matter of finding a new home because he'd accepted a job ninety minutes away and commuting like that wasn't an option, it was a slow-motion collapse.

We talked in chunks that could survive interruption, because my hands could only last minutes in the freezer mitts before my fingers started screaming. My toes could take twice as long. Scott managed the socks—on, off, on again—while I tried to keep my mouth cold with frozen grapes, my mouth-sore prevention trick turned fleshy chemical experiment.

I lasted three minutes. Five on a heroic day. The mitts came off, fingers red and stinging, and then—because chemo is nothing if not repetitive—they went right back on.

Once Taxotere finished, I got my body parts back. The games came out. They were chosen with care: small table-friendly, light thinking, no strategy required—something my brain could do while it slowly turned to mush.

Cytoxan dripped for an hour and the metallic taste peaked right then—tea, grapes, tongue—everything with the faint tang of a battery. I drank warm green tea in tiny sips, mostly to remind my throat it still knew how to swallow. Sometimes we watched stand-up or a short show. Sometimes Scott answered emails while I closed my eyes and tried to meditate through it.

At some point the fluids did what fluids do. I'd unwrap myself from the blanket, shove my feet back into shoes, switch the drip to battery mode, unplug from the wall, and shuffle to the restroom pushing my IV pole like a reluctant dance partner. "Stage 1" didn't mention the part where you become a person who schedules bathroom breaks around a drip.

The nurses were good—welcoming, generous with snacks and normal conversation. They asked about the kids. We asked about their lives, too, because it helped to remember the world still had other topics.

Four hours in, everything had been tended to. We'd head home with the same two backpacks. I never felt like I brought the same body back. I would be ready for the nap that wasn't a luxury so much as a medical requirement.

Cancer Gone Public

I was told my hair would fall out. Nothing was said about how much it hurts first. My scalp felt ablaze for days before a single strand let go. Then came the evidence—on my pillow, in my hands, clinging to sweaters like static confession.

One sunny afternoon in those first weeks, Scott pulled out the clippers. We set up in the bathroom. He used a number-two guard and moved carefully. We joked about matching bald heads and making it our holiday card. Dark humor became our oxygen.

Afterward, we took a selfie and sent it to the kids, scattered across Colorado, Iowa, and Utah. One texted that his coworkers said I looked gorgeous. Another sent hearts so many times the screen lagged. One walked into the kitchen, looked me squarely in the eye, and said, "It's really freaky to see you like this. I appreciate you wearing hats around the house so you're not traumatizing me unnecessarily." As if I picked beanies for his comfort and not because my skull had discovered a draft.

The truth? Shaving didn't make me cry. Weirdly, it felt like relief—an honest head for an honest season. The aftermath was louder. Hair loss made cancer public. Strangers' eyes stalled in grocery aisles. I tried not to look back. Most days I didn't go anywhere; being immunocompromised is its own winter. At the clinic, I was one of many, which was both solace and erasure.

I'd considered a cooling cap, but the odds weren't in my favor and my tolerance for sitting in ice was zero. No regrets.

Accumulation

By cycle two, the clinic smell could turn my stomach before anyone said hello. By cycle three, I stopped believing I'd "bounce back." By cycle four, I would've signed any contract that ended with: no more. Chemo didn't happen once. It happened again. And again. And the "again" was the point.

Chemo took plenty with it: taste, fingerprints (who knew?), time. My tongue felt like sandpaper. Water tasted metallic. Fatigue settled in at the cellular level.

Most mornings, I'd make it halfway down the stairs and sit—hands gripping the banister, forehead on my forearm—negotiating gravity. Then the rest of the stairs. Then the chair at the bottom. Then the kitchen. Then tea. Warm tea replaced coffee. It was the only thing my mouth trusted. Wrapping my fingers around the mug was a momentary truce—evidence I still had a body with a job to do.

I was grateful for chemo and furious about it at the same time.

The Devil Wears Neulasta

Neulasta is marketed like an invisible shield: boosts white blood cells! Lowers infection risk! What the pamphlet doesn't say is that my first dose would find me on the bedroom floor like a felled tree.

It comes in a plastic pod that sticks to your belly and auto-injects twenty-seven hours after chemo. Cute, in an animated short. In real life, the green light blinked, there was a click, and my body went to DEFCON puke. Cold sweat. Flat spin. Nausea like a freight train.

I went down onto the hardwood and rolled on my side (aspiration prevention: the one skill set I wanted not to use at home), and stayed there thirty minutes wrestling with mortality through walnut-colored wood grain. This was the nectar of Satan himself.

After that, we changed the plan: half-dose, slower delivery, at the infusion center with eyes on me. Even half-dosed and slow, it still felt like shaking hands with the devil.

Bald and Beloved

Two friends sent the best chemo gift: a box with tabloids, candy cigarettes, foot balm, and pièce de résistance—photoshopped images of themselves, gloriously bald, beaming like starlets.

I laughed so hard I almost peed. I still have those pictures. Love plus absurdity is a treatment plan.

Identity Whiplash and Micro-Mercies

Appointments cluttered the calendar. At the hospital, I used to be the one explaining. Now I was the one being explained to.

Once, a nurse who knew me from the hospital did a small double-take—caught it with Olympic speed—and then got kind. Too kind. I wanted to say, "I know. It's weird when the person with the badge has a bracelet instead."

People offered everything from smoothies to crystals, playlists to a drive-by drop of soup in a pot I didn't recognize and have not seen since. The useful things were small and unglamorous: a neighbor who hauled my trash cans when Scott was away, a friend texting "doorstep" and leaving without knocking, Scott laying out morning meds beside a full water glass like a daily brief.

I told Scott I wanted to label my bald head LIMITED EDITION. He said it would ruin my market positioning. We were insufferable and deeply in love.

Side Effects: The Uncategorizable

Some things don't fit neatly into drug sheets. The itch that woke me at 3 a.m. The way my hands acted like every jar required advanced negotiations. The moments when thoughts felt like migrating birds I could almost, not quite, track across the sky.

And the day I tried to wear jeans and my skin protested. The denim felt like a mesh of fiberglass and regret.

Food went sideways. Crackers became the enemy. Tea a friend. Ginger, my therapist. I built a small altar to blandness: rice, bananas, broth. We tried everything the internet suggested short of witchcraft (jury's still out).

For mouth sores, I swished a magic mouthwash that tasted like old garden hose dipped in sugar. It worked. I also developed a little superstition of glaring at the bottle every time. It worked less. It still mattered.

What "Stage 1" Doesn't Say

Stage 1 is the diagnosis that makes people exhale. I don't blame them. The world loves a story with a reassuring narrative: the crisis passes, the body bounces back, the credits roll.

But credits don't roll in the infusion chair. They don't wake to bone-deep ache. They don't carry hair to the trash like a small funeral. "Early" is true and also incomplete. My Stage 1 came with asterisks, footnotes, and fine print. It was complicated as hell.

Eventually I made a glossary:

- Stage 1A: early stage, yes; also aggressive biology.
- Oncotype 37: the number that flipped the table.
- TC chemo: a Suffering Bastard cocktail—no bartender, no returns.
- Neulasta: necessary evil; please hand-hold.

That glossary wasn't for anyone else. It was a shorthand for me—a way to keep the story from unraveling every time someone said, "At least it's Stage 1."

Small Rebellions

I bought a ridiculous scarf in tomato red and sea-glass teal. I wore giant hooped earrings to nowhere. I learned the precise temperature at which broth becomes a small miracle (I'm not saying it was sacred, but damn if it wasn't saving me).

One day my eyebrows started to bail. I drew them right back on. I considered it art.

I said no to unsolicited miracle cures with all the politeness of a brick. I said yes to naps like they were a graduate seminar. I started blocking off whole afternoons on the calendar and labeling them Do Not Attempt Heroics. If rest was going to be my side job, it was getting office hours.

Tig Notaro showed up on my couch again. I didn't need the whole set—just the audacity. She told the truth and dared me not to laugh. I answered back: "Fine. I'll laugh and cry. Multitasking is my only sport."

The Last Laugh

Somewhere between chemo cycles, I found myself laughing—really laughing—at something objectively dumb (I believe our cat rolled off the couch unintentionally and then postured like it never happened). The sound startled me. It also returned me to myself. Chemo hadn't taken everything.

By the end of that season, I had a killer scarf collection, a head that could frighten a pharmacy line, and a sense of humor that survived contact with reality. Stage 1, sure—but it brought the whole circus. Monkeys, too.

I won't pretend there was a lesson in it. There was persistence. There was love. There were small, ludicrous gifts—bald glamour shots and candy cigarettes. There were mornings I made it from bed to chair and called it a triumph. There were nights I laid a hand on my strange new chest and said, "Okay. We still belong to each other."

Stage 1, sure. With footnotes.

Chemo didn't make me brave. It made me honest.

Survivorship: Terms and Conditions Apply

The Fine Print

Survival is not a before-and-after photo. It's not a pink ribbon tied neatly around your life or a bell rung in triumph with nothing but clear skies ahead. It's not the last page of a chapter.

Survival is messy. Chronic. Full of caveats.

It looks like wearing compression sleeves on a 97-degree day because cancer treatment rearranged the plumbing and my arm balloons by lunch. It looks like juggling follow-ups and PET scans like they're normal errands. Groceries. Scanxiety. Car wash. Physical therapy. Repeat.

It looks like wondering if every headache is a wire humming toward something you don't want to name. Like being grateful to still be here while also furious your body turned on you. "Early" didn't mean spared. Survivorship includes insurance skirmishes, new meds with fine-print side effects, and sensory flashbacks that ambush you at Sprouts—like the day my mouth filled with metal so sharply I could smell it, just from passing the grapes in produce.

It looks like watching the world carry on while you still feel like a half-built structure—scaffolding up, wires exposed, nothing fully secured. It's hearing "strong" and "brave" when what people mean is, I care. I don't know what to say. Please don't make me look at the edge.

And then there are the people who say, "Whatever you need, I'm here," and vanish like a bad magic trick.

But survival also comes with a kind of clarity no gratitude journal can teach. A no-bullshit lens that strips away the unnecessary and sharpens what matters.

I know who my people are now. They showed up to help us move—they stacked dishes and wiped shelves. They touched up paint, carried boxes. They brought meals that were frozen, labeled, chemo-friendly, and thoughtfully bland. Exactly what I needed.

I built boundaries out of necessity, and they held. No toxic compliments about my appearance. No shame over scars. No hiding my port to make others comfortable. I kept my T-Rex arms and my sense of humor. Both helped me heal.

I learned something else: I can carry more than I ever wanted to prove. And I'll never use the word "early" to make someone else's diagnosis sound easier than it is.

Minimal Stage, Maximal Upheaval

Stage 1A wasn't the story. It was the opening line. It meant pulling the emergency brake on my life and then steering through smoke.

My career path stalled. I needed more help from my kids than I could give them. My relationship with Scott tilted into survival mode—he was steady; I became high-maintenance in every category: physical, emotional, cognitive. One surgery became two, then more. Chemo, then endocrine therapy, the door kept opening, each time revealing some new indignity or obligation.

Stairs became negotiations. My muscles softened. T-shirts gave way to button-ups because my arms wouldn't lift over my head. I didn't just lose my boobs; I lost freedom. No grocery carts, no vacuuming. No walking the dog. Energy had to be rationed like a rare currency.

The kitchen reorganized itself around my limitations. Plates and bowls came down to the counter; the cheese drawer became prime real estate in the fridge; coffee turned collaborative.

One morning I decided to do it myself—because I missed being a person who could complete a basic task without calling a committee meeting. I pulled out a stool to reach the water reservoir and refilled it. When I tried to angle it back in, my shoulder said no. Not pain exactly—more like a hard stop.

I tried again, slower, jaw clenched, pretending effort could negotiate anatomy. The tank wobbled. Water sloshed. My throat tightened with that particular flavor of humiliation: This is such a stupid thing to need help with.

"Scott," I called, casual on purpose. "Can you—just for a second?"

He stepped in, did the same motion I'd just failed at, and it clicked into place like it had been waiting for his hands. No commentary. No pity. Just competence.

"There," he said.

I swallowed the lump that wanted to become a sermon about independence. Coffee didn't turn collaborative. I had to.

"Nothing heavier than a gallon of milk," they said. I measured my days in liters and spoons.

Even the dog had to adapt. We sent him to my dad's house right after the mastectomy. Part retriever, part wrecking ball—too risky for surgical drains. The short stay stretched to almost five weeks—first my recovery, then my dad's pre-planned road trip. A dog's dream: new smells, lakes, endless backseat naps. When he finally came home, he shadowed me room to room, watching my feet like they might betray me. Loyal, slightly miffed, and—like me—a little lost.

At PT, I learned how to coax range of motion from stubborn fascia. Wall slides. Wand lifts. Lymphatic strokes I could do in the shower while pretending it was a spa. My therapist cheered the moment my right arm climbed past shoulder height. I cried the first time I could fasten my seatbelt without strategy.

Strong Enough to Perform It

The survivor narrative: triumphant posts in pink font. "I kicked cancer's ass" in acrylic block letters. It's easier to root for someone who looks brave and sounds like they were born to win. It's polished, uplifting, and easily digestible.

Support arrived in waves—pink boxing gloves from my mom's friend, messages wrapped in condolences and compliments: You're so strong. You've got this. Overnight, I was branded a warrior. I didn't want to fight. I didn't want to be brave.

That wasn't my story. Mine was a diagnosis that kept evolving, a slow unraveling of certainty, one complication into the next.

I just didn't want to die.

To survive, I performed strength for the comfort of others. Women are trained for this: be it all, do it all. Even sick, keep caregiving. Keep smiling. Keep making other people okay with your reality.

I kept that performance up through surgery, through the first rounds of chemo, through the spring. But eight months in, the façade crumbled. I was stuck, emotionally flatlined. Not leading my life, just surviving inside it. I started ketamine-assisted therapy. My first session cracked something open.

I drifted through geometric folds and canyon walls until a small bird appeared. It looked up and chirped once, asking to be lifted. I picked it up. It wasn't hurt; it wasn't mine to fix. I held it to the light and released it: It's time to fly.

The journey turned inward. I met my cancer cells in color: amber, blood orange, focused and quiet. Not evil—just doing their job. And they were mine. Driven, rebellious, aggressively productive—creating something strange and misguided with conviction. A rogue version of my ambition.

Later, I knew: the bird was everyone I'd been carrying. People I tried to protect; people who leaned on me like a dock. They could fly. Letting them go made space for someone I'd ignored entirely: me.

Not the version performing strength. The real one—the one who needed tenderness, rest, and permission to be cared for without offering anything back.

If I loved myself, how could I go to war against my own creation?

The Cancer Pacifist

The phrase arrived like a lifeline—maybe from a forum, maybe from the ether—but it stuck: cancer pacifist.

Being a cancer pacifist means rejecting war metaphors.

The first time someone told me to "fight," I nodded and felt my whole body say no. I wasn't a soldier. I wasn't "battling." I wasn't fighting cancer any more than I was fighting myself. I was healing—sometimes gracefully, sometimes chaotically—but never violently.

I've never felt at war with my body. I've felt confused by it. Betrayed, yes. But also in awe. Those cells—even the ones gone feral—were trying to survive. They were built from me, fed by me, patterned after me.

Pacifism meant choosing compassion over conquest. Being present for grief and fear instead of pushing them out with platitudes. Rejecting forced positivity. Reclaiming language that reflected reality.

It gave me space to be honest—with Scott, with my body, with myself. Self-compassion instead of self-blame. Humor instead of hostility. Gratitude instead of glory. Permission to make meaning in the mess, not just in the aftermath.

Being a cancer pacifist didn't mean surrendering to illness. It meant surrendering to healing.

And that felt like the bravest thing I could do.

Invisible Weights

Fearless isn't the right word. I felt fear—just not of cancer itself. I feared what it would take: roles, rhythms, worth.

As my confidence grew in one area—treatment decisions—I kept turning that strength outward. Reassurance became my currency. I spent it freely. I offered calm I didn't feel. I became ballast for people who couldn't stomach seeing me adrift.

Asking for help? I didn't know how. Staying busy serving others worked like bubble wrap over panic. The double-edged sword of competence: you hold so much that no one thinks to ask if it's breaking you.

Underneath, there was an ache. Asking—even to water the plants—felt like confessing failure. In the twisted math of internalized expectations, that made me a less-than-capable woman.

Exhaustion followed. Guilt. A strange invisibility. I was the center of attention, rarely seen. People praised resilience and missed grief. They didn't notice the depressive thoughts behind the default smile, the rage over having so little control.

I felt guilt for not doing it all—especially with teenagers living their own weather systems in our orbit.

Proof arrived one night when my phone lit up with my kid's name from college.

"I had a panic attack today," they said, like they were reporting a quiz grade.

"Oh, kiddo." I sat up. "Are you okay right now?"

A pause. Then: "Yeah. I didn't call you earlier because… you have cancer."

I held the phone with both hands, useless with distance. I wanted to do the only things mothers do on instinct: pull them into a hug, listen, fix the air in the room. Instead I said, "I'm here. Tell me what happened," and tried not to sound like I was borrowing someone else's voice.

That's what I mean by invisible weight. Not chores. Not dinner. The slow grief of watching roles shift while everyone pretends it's temporary. I wasn't just missing plans. I was missing my place.

And then came the shame—when I asked others for help with things I believed should still be mine. And, yes, resentment. Watching other people move through their days unpaused—vacations, promotions, dinner parties. I was happy for them. I also envied their ease—the way they moved in the kitchen, stood at a stove, held a conversation like it cost nothing.

My limited range of motion made that impossible. During chemo, even seeing people in restaurant booths could gut me. My immune system couldn't risk public spaces. And even if it could, the mouth sores and nausea would've stolen the joy anyway.

It wasn't about missing dinner. It was about missing living.

Faith and Friction

In the weeks after ketamine, I kept trying to practice the only thing that felt true: presence. Not solutions. Not slogans. Just showing up and staying. It wasn't mystical. It was daily—letting people love me imperfectly, letting myself be cared for without performing "fine."

And then the prayers came.

Accepting them was complicated.

Prayer, I realized, is another dialect of uncertainty—how people reach for meaning when they can't fix what's happening.

"Jesus will lead the way" didn't land gently. It felt hollow. Sometimes intrusive. I knew people meant well. Their intentions were good. But their comfort didn't fit in my body. I made peace with the unknown a long time ago. Agnosticism has never been a wound for me. The ache didn't come from a silent sky; it came from the assumption that I needed the heavens to speak.

I wanted to be gracious. To honor care without betraying belief. That's hard while surviving. Existential nuance is hard when the daily goal is: make it through. When someone said they were praying, I thanked them—politely, automatically. And sometimes I thought, What the hell—maybe their God can pull something off.

Trauma invites its siblings. Old baggage joins the pile. The prayers became packages of meaning that didn't quite belong to me. I brought them to therapy with the rest.

Over time, they softened. The sting faded. I understood the prayers weren't really for me; they were offerings—extensions of faith. I can respect that, even if I don't share it.

For me, "Sending love" always meant more. "Holding space." "Thinking of you." "I'm here."

Those were the terms I could accept: presence over prayer. Witness over intervention.

Tenderness as a Practice

Survival isn't radiant, packaged, or especially pink. It isn't a glossy redemption arc or a steady climb upward. It's scar tissue and side effects. It's waking exhausted and showing up anyway.

It's not fearless. It's tenderness.

Even when it hurts. Especially when it hurts.

Because tenderness is where the good stuff lives: love, meaning, honesty, connection. Not the slogans or ribbons or deft sound bites, but the raw, breaking truth of what it takes to keep going.

That's what I'm choosing. Again and again.

Survival doesn't follow a script. It doesn't need to. It isn't linear. There's no well-marked trail with cairns and signage. No guidebook.

It unfolds—like the paper fortune tellers we made in grade school. Fingers moving underneath, flipping and folding, revealing answers you didn't choose. Pick a color, a number, a direction—you still don't know what's coming next. Sometimes it says, You'll marry your crush. Sometimes, You'll fall in the mud. Either way, the hands underneath are already moving.

And me? Not fearless. Not a fighter.

Just human.

Choosing tenderness.

The terms are never final. The forecast is mostly "maybe."

And tomorrow's chapter has a name: uncertainty.

The Language of Uncertainty

Sometimes the fog is where the truth lives.

The thing about cancer is that it's saturated with uncertainty. One day you're answering texts and baking cookies; the next, life takes a hard left without signaling. Whatever confidence I'd built in my tolerance for disruption dissolved on contact. Tumors arrive like uninvited houseguests and suddenly I'm living by the meter of chemo: drips, labs, naps, repeat. Uncertainty stamped itself on the inside of everything: nothing is promised.

When the Language Betrays You

Four rounds of chemo: complete. Five months held the whole spectacle—diagnosis, mastectomy, port in, chemo, port out. Post-infusion, I walked into my six-week follow-up believing "after" had begun. We set out the next step like adults planning a remodel: aromatase inhibitors to starve estrogen, the accelerant I didn't ask for. The clinic drew tumor markers "for baseline."

They came back slightly elevated. Huh.

We repeated them a week later. Higher. Fuck.

My oncologist was baffled. This wasn't the script. "Let's get a PET."

Tumor markers aren't supposed to be a prophecy, but mine were trying to become one.

Waiting rooms have a particular silence. Not peaceful—more like hush braided with bargaining. I knew the climate: the sound of shoes on linoleum, the faint television no one watches, the eternal scent of hospital hand foam. It was my first PET. I went alone—still untrained in dread.

They call it scanxiety, a word too cutesy that offends the gravity of what it names. It's not worry; it's anguish. Your body rehearses every worst-case scenario you've ever tried to out-think. You rehearse grief before the cue—heart hammering—while the machine clicks with no known tempo. The tech wrapped me in a warm blanket. "Stay still," he said, as if stillness were a thing that could be willed. By the time the table slid me out, I'd mentally drafted my eulogy twice and edited for tone. Irrational, and also not.

The next evening, I wasn't expecting bad news. That's the trick of it—I'd been compliant, busy stitching my life back together. The oncologist called with that neutral, careful voice trained to sound calm while implosion occurs. I put her on speaker and found Scott's hand.

"The result of your PET scan is positive."

Language is a minefield. In medicine, positive is bad and negative is good. Unremarkable is the compliment you actually want. Stable sounds like you won—but it just means not worse. Progression is a dirty word. Clear margins reads like salvation. Overnight, my emotional life was tethered to adjectives and tense. I lived in the grammar between things: not cured, not terminal. Not fine, not falling apart. Suspended between parts of speech.

Case Study, Human

Words reached me as if underwater, floating up slowly: three lymph nodes lit. Two in the axilla, one tucked against the chest wall. Cancer confirmed. Biopsy next.

I no longer needed an escort to interventional radiology; I could've given a tour. The nurse asked why I was there and I heard my voice say, "Recurrence," like the word belonged to someone else. Secretly I wanted a clerical error. A fluke. A plot twist.

The pathology refused orderliness. The first samples were small and contradictory. Plot twist granted. We did a second biopsy for more tissue. Results still didn't match each other—or my original diagnosis. One node was ER positive, PR negative. Another read triple negative. My original tumors were ER positive, PR positive. What the actual hell? The chest node lounged worryingly close to a nerve bundle you'd really like cancer to leave alone. "Might not be removable," someone said in the polite voice people use when looking away.

My surgeon took it on anyway. She asked her team for prayers. It's not the pre-op note you crave, but I didn't have a better theology to offer.

Five mediastinal nodes came out—four cancerous. Twelve axillary—three cancerous. The PET had glowed at three; the scalpel discovered seven. Worse than expected by any numbering system. "What does this mean?" I asked. She sent me back to oncology for interpretation —results delivered, meaning deferred.

Recovery was brutal. My right arm went on strike. No coffee cup, no steering wheel, no deodorant without strategy. Any wrong move and I risked internal bleeding. A drain dangled from my armpit like a bored ornament and produced nothing. This wasn't pain so much as a geography lesson: border redrawn, roads closed, detours enforced. Mourning movement, mourning ease, mourning the illusion of control.

The New Math

Here is another truth: cancer isn't just illness; it's middle management. Medication schedules, appointment grids, prescriptions with personalities. Frozen grapes, compression sleeves, sitz baths, laxatives, gentle PT. I became the project manager of my own body—tracking metrics, identifying bottlenecks, escalating to specialists. Spreadsheets, timers, pill sorters. Even a "good" day required paperwork. Rest became a task. Hygiene, a strategy. Survival, administration.

Then came the updated plan—the kind of paragraph you recite with your eyes on your shoes because meeting someone's gaze makes the words too real to carry. The oncologist spoke, and I translated the data into the currency of my actual life.

"Treat the first cancer and the new cancer at the same time," she said. Internal: As if they were two unruly tenants in a building I no longer owned. I wondered if they'd fight each other for space, or if I was just the neutral ground being burned so neither could win.

"Endocrine therapy on pause." Internal: A temporary reprieve from the chemical menopause, but the safety gate was swinging wide open. The estrogen I'd spent months trying to starve was suddenly back on the menu.

"Time for a new port." Internal: My skin was already a map of old wounds and scar tissue. I pictured the surgeon searching for a patch of virgin territory to stitch the plastic disc into. Fine, I thought. Install the hardware. Upgrade the infrastructure.

"Four months Carbo/Gemzar IV chemo with every third week off." Internal: A schedule that pretended to include mercy.

"Neulasta." Internal: Back like a bad sequel—bone pain on standby.

"Immunotherapy layered in for nine months." Internal: A full pregnancy of medicine.

"Then radiation. Daily. Six and a half weeks." Internal: Thirty-three drives, thirty-three days of blue light and ozone.

"Then six months of oral chemo." Internal: The kitchen-cabinet metronome that never lets you forget.

"Then likely a revision surgery." Internal: Because radiation doesn't leave tissue without a receipt. The skin would become wood; the breast would become a memory of a memory.

I sat there, mentally updating the spreadsheet of my life. I was no longer a person; I was a series of billable hours and biological reactions. I was a project to be managed, a bottleneck to be cleared. Survival didn't feel like a victory; it felt like administration.

Digesting all this was confusing. I delivered it to family like a shipping estimate. I sounded soothing, which is what numbness wears to work. I booked acupuncture, called the dentist, canceled the oophorectomy, resumed PT, scheduled therapy. I read studies I didn't want to understand and forum threads I'd promised to avoid. Triple-negative cancer is known for its unrelenting aggression. The recurrence risk is elevated day one and peaks at year three; then drops dramatically, overnight. It's like a jagged ridgeline no one is equipped to hike.

Meanwhile, my brain scribbled in the margins: Will I keep up with school through another course of chemo? Is respiratory therapy now a closed door? Do I sink years and tuition into a new path if I don't trust the calendar? Five-year stats barged in uninvited. I named five years a shoreline—something to aim for when you can't see the horizon.

Will I work again? What does working even mean now? How do I live like it counts without sprinting myself into dust?

Phrases lodged and stayed like burrs in a sock: supported loneliness; impressively battered; grateful upheaval.

Inventory

There is a moment—in chemo bathrooms, in parking lots, at the edge of a bed—you take inventory of your life like it's a pantry before a blizzard.

I had a husband who kept showing up with broth and soft competence. Kids who offered jokes precisely when jokes were not possible. Friends who texted pictures of rivers and dogs and the sky when language failed. A house mid-move and a dog who learned to adjust his joy to my surgical drains. I had a body that was both furious and faithful. I had a mind that could read itself into a corner and then ask for help.

I also had a head that was almost hair again, bristly like a field in late winter. I shaved the last stubborn stubble and decided if round two wanted me, I'd show up bald on purpose. It felt like choosing something in a world that kept choosing me first.

Adverse Events (A Love Story)

Cycle one included Gemzar. Within hours my skin composed an opera. A rash bloomed across my belly, chest, neck—an emergency flare written in red. It wasn't surface itch; it was deeper than language, a slow-motion scream below the dermis. I sent photos to the oncologist: "Uh… Houston, we have a problem."

"Benadryl. Oatmeal baths. Keep cool," came the answer, clinical and kind.

So I steeped like a human teabag and tried not to crawl out of my body. At the clinic: "You've had a severe allergic reaction to Gemzar," delivered with the passive tone that announces tornadoes and airline delays. Not normal, not dangerous—the shrug that would become the caption for too much of what followed.

After one week off to calm the skin, we stayed the course with a heroic pre-med of IV Benadryl before every infusion. It didn't knock me out. It did the opposite. It lit my nerves on fire—frantic, bone-deep restlessness that turned my legs to iron vises. I learned to stare at a spot on the wall and lengthen time. I sat, endlessly adjusting my weight, and rode the drip.

Put it in the margin: not normal, not dangerous, just miserable.

How to Carry a Day

Here is how I carried a day in that season:

Up before the house due to insomnia, because silence is a kind of medicine. Tea becomes ceremony—a small cup, lukewarm so my mouth can tolerate it. Check the portal against my better judgment. Label the pill box because labels are a fragile kind of safety. Stretch scar tissue with the patience of a gardener coaxing vines along a trellis. Text a friend a photo of the morning sky and let their reply stand in for courage.

Drive to the clinic with a water bottle rolling around on the passenger floor. Greet every phlebotomist by name and pretend I don't know their vein preference. Thank the nurse who remembers where my favorite blanket lives. Sit in the tan chair, the chair so many bodies have warmed. Watch the IV pump blink its small green promises. Think of nothing. Think of everything.

On the way home, listen to my liked songs playlist. In the driveway, stay in the car long enough to finish a song. Walk inside like a person who meant to come back.

Evidence of Living

Uncertainty isn't just a feeling; it is architecture. It builds rooms in your day you didn't plan for. A nook for crying where no one can see you. A shelf for research articles you shouldn't read after 9 p.m. A drawer where you keep the hand lotion that reminds you of camping trips, because memory is both comfort and ache. A spot in the closet for the compression sleeves, absurdly ordinary.

By then I had developed a personal grammar of medical speech. "Probably" means no one knows yet. "For now" means your relief is on a timer. "We'll see" is both honest and insufficient. I learned which adjectives deserve tears and which only merit a highlighter. I learned that surgeons speak in nouns and oncologists in verbs. I learned the portal will get a nickname whether you want it to or not; it becomes loved and distrusted all at once.

There were still glimmers. The dog's soft insistence on being at my feet. The way Scott could make cookies exactly right and place them in front of me without commentary. The day I removed the seat belt padding—another emotional burden removed. The neighbor who left a bag of lemons and a sticky note that just said, "More light."

Given: A renewed ability to say no without apology. A ruthless filter for what matters. A small, stubborn joy in ordinary rituals.

Taken: Range of motion. Spontaneity. The particular freedom of planning something for months from now and assuming your body will cooperate. Rooms that used to be safe—restaurants, classrooms, clinics—suddenly requiring new rules.

Given: People who show up with enchiladas absent of all traces of spice, just the way I needed them to be. A therapist who could hold silence without stuffing it full of platitudes. A sense of humor that survived chemo and learned to wink on the way to the bathroom.

Taken: Time. A type of innocence I didn't know was there until it was gone.

What We Told Each Other

When Scott and I learned about the next year of treatment, we treated the plan like a complicated itinerary: flights, layovers, a couple of questionable connections. He asked where he needed to be and when. "Here," I said, because the answer never changed.

Telling the kids was different. They were in the kitchen, fridge door open, searching for salsa. I said the thing I had to say and watched faces lift, then set—quick-drying concrete. "Again?" "Yes." We stood there with the cold air reaching our knees. Later, Max texted me a meme that was objectively dumb. It was perfect.

Telling my dad broke something tender. He is a practical man who fixes things with tools. There is no wrench for this. I started to talk, then sobbed, while we hugged. Silence that is not empty but full of whatever love can do when it can't do anything.

Bodies keep their own dictionaries. I learned to name sensations without marrying them. I learned the difference between spiraling and looking ahead. I learned that certain fluorescent lights could make me nauseated before the appointment even began.

And the mind, a loyal archivist, collected everything: standardized uptake values and odds ratios, discharge instructions and half-heard reassurance. I became good at separating data from doom. I became better at closing the laptop.

Practice, Not Proof

People sometimes talk about uncertainty as a test of faith. It never felt like that to me. It felt like practice. A practice of attention and restraint. Of knowing when to research and when to watch a dumb show. Of admitting I was scared and letting that be a sentence, not a performance review. Of asking, "How is today?" and letting today answer without forecasting tomorrow.

I practiced tenderness the way you practice scales. Not because it was noble, but because it's hard. Because my body responded better to softness than to war.

The language of uncertainty is a way of living. It's probably and for now and we'll see, spoken earnestly. It's learning which words deserve your tears and which only deserve a pen stroke. It's naming the shapes you can see and leaving space for the ones you can't. It's letting love in even while you're triaging.

The fog doesn't always lift. You learn to walk in it.

And when the plan expands again—chemo overlapping with something new; a specialist added like a surprise character—you carry the map you didn't want and redraw it in the margins. You keep a ledger that will never balance and write grace in the notes column. You stand at the clinic window, watch the late light catch dust in the air, and decide that being here is both enough and everything.

Next: the daily ritual that burns and benefits, the machine that hums like a threat pretending to be routine, the season of lotion and lasers. But first, a breath.

Quiet Burn

The Flatirons watched me do it.

Beautiful. Stoic. Iconic. They were a stone audience to my 8:30 a.m. ritual—arrive, undress, align, hold still—five days a week while winter rehearsed its gray. From my bedroom deck in Longmont, I could trace that serrated line, then drive straight toward it until the mountains filled the windshield, Foothills Hospital tucked into their lap. They saw all my arrivals and departures, the way the season couldn't decide between fall and winter and, frankly, neither could I.

The Consult

Radiation added a new specialist to the roster: the doctor who would burn me on purpose and call it care. He was exacting in a way that felt like safety. We talked fields and fractions; the breast bed and the regional nodes; timelines and side effects.

"We start a few weeks after chemo ends," he said. "Thirty-three treatments, including a boost."

It sounded straightforward. In a body with a life, daily means daily. Radiation doesn't negotiate. He added the standard comfort—"Most people tolerate it well"—the way clinicians lay a calm hand on an avalanche. I nodded. I've learned that my tolerance is not the same as my body's.

Simulation

Late November. All the leaves had dropped, and the sky had gone to stainless steel. Mapping day felt like an odd rite of passage. I lay on the CT table molding a cradle for my shoulders, head, and back. Arms overhead, chin angled just so while green lasers quartered me into precise geography. The techs were friendly and meticulous: "A touch to your left…hold…you're doing great."

They drew on me with Sharpie, then marked three pinprick tattoos—blue freckles with jobs. I asked how my skin would change with radiation. "You'll glow," one tech said, "only socially." We laughed the way you laugh when everyone in the room is fluent in gallows humor.

I drove home with a latte I'd made in my kitchen—my throat tolerated warm milk better than café bravado—and queued an alt-rock playlist I've been overplaying since 2011. Ritual, meet ritual.

Twenty Minutes to Incandescence

Mid-December, the burns began invisibly—first as composition. Radiation became a commute. I parked in the same radiation-patient spot, grabbed my water bottle and the zip bag of creams. The room was colder than strictly necessary, which I think was to keep bodies obedient. The table was cool under my shoulder blades; the cradle clicked into the notch my bones learned by heart. Ordinary breathing became a skill set: soft, shallow, steady.

"About ten minutes," the techs would say, and step out. The door sealed with the submarine finality that tells you a machine is about to do something you can't. The gantry swung overhead like a benevolent planet. I kept my orbit. Buzz. Click. Pause. Red alignment dots speckled the air. The room always smelled faintly of warmed plastic and ozone, the way new electronics do when they first wake up. I tried to think about nothing and then, predictably, thought about everything. They came back, rotated the arc, adjusted my cradle angle. I tried not to assign meaning to the rotations, as if the machine had tea leaves to read.

Daily makes you efficient. On a good morning I was in and out in twenty minutes, the Flatirons smirking as I drove home, coffee cooling in the cup holder, music loud enough to make my sternum buzz. The mountains never answered back. That was their gift.

Winter, Wearing Fire

By the second week, the entry field blushed. The next week, it pinked. Then red. The air outside was crisp enough to sting; the mountains were gray against a silver sky. The disparity between my glowing chest and the winter air felt like a cosmic joke. It was perfectly timed, though—the heat trapped in my skin meant I could walk from clinic to car without a coat. A sweater felt like a brick; a coat, a personal assault. The instant relief of cold air on scorched skin was followed by instant tightness, the way a puddle skins over when the temperature drops. My body was suddenly full of weather.

The first thing I did at home every day was shower, lukewarm at best. Gentle suds to wash away the baked-in clinic smell. Then Scott's hands spreading lotion and calendula across my back in long, careful strokes. We didn't need to talk about radiation; there wasn't anything to say that would make sense over the quiet.

Wardrobe became engineering. I couldn't wear a bra—too raw. Couldn't wear nipple covers—also too raw. Bulky sweaters and sweatshirts were too heavy. It was, regrettably, nipples-under-T-shirt season: Christmas, New Year's, all of it. Great for a sexy date night; less great when your stepkids are in the kitchen asking about finals.

I missed the luxury of a fire, the weightless heat on the side of your face when you lean in to roast nothing in particular. Even coffee out with friends lost its charm—the heat and acidity were too much for a throat that was catching the edge of the beam. Concerts were worst of all: I could stand in the back, sure, but I couldn't belt the chorus or dance without thinking about seams and straps and the latitude of my pain. I love concerts. Radiation burned that love into a complicated shape.

Supported Loneliness

People assume daily treatment comes with daily company. It doesn't. The staff was lovely; the routine, precise; the conversations efficient by design. Radiation is an intimacy with a machine. You learn the faces of the techs, who tells a clean joke, whose "you're doing great" lands without tipping you into tears. Friends texted; Scott kept the meds straight and made warm tapioca pudding when my throat went raspy. Mostly, I wanted to slip under this wave and let it pass. Supported loneliness is exactly what it sounds like: held and alone at the same time.

So I built micro-rituals to carry the macro beam:

- Park nose-out so the sun warms the dashboard, not the seatback.
- Two deep breaths before opening the car door.
- Always take the changing room on the right; its bench is friendlier, its robes less scratchy.
- Thank the machine. Quietly, so as not to worry the humans. They saw a linear accelerator; I saw a co-conspirator. We had a deal: it would burn the bad cells, and I would hold still enough to let it.
- Smother lotion before a shirt touches me, sip water after.
- Loud music all the way home.

These weren't cures. They were small places to stand.

The Violence of Quiet

Radiation sells itself as cumulative, which is its elegance and its trick. At first: nothing. Then a hint of color where, in winter, none should be. Pretty, almost. Then oversaturated, grotesque, tender in a way that felt smarter than metaphor. My back burned worse than my front—a geometry problem I didn't think to solve. The field wrapped farther than my imagination, and my throat—caught at the edge—went raw. By then I had a routine: lotion and calendula by day, Aquaphor at night, applied with the tenderness of someone frosting a very angry cake. I sorted shirts by seam betrayal. I slept hard and woke tired. Fatigue arrived like sea smoke on a lake—biting, sure of itself, disrespectful of plans. I could go from upright to horizontal in the time it takes a shower to warm up.

The machine kept humming. The techs kept aligning me to millimeters. I kept showing up. This is the violence of quiet: the thing that saves you is also the thing that asks for your surface, every day, while you're still trying to be a person who answers texts.

Meanwhile, immunotherapy continued its drumbeat—every twenty-one days. This time in a grey chair and a view of Long's Peak in the distance. It is a particular strangeness to be burned and infused at once—physics from the outside, chemistry from the inside, a coordinated pincer action against cells that were mine and misbehaving. Lists were loyal in a way feelings weren't. I let logistics drive when emotion fishtailed.

Last Call

The last week felt ceremonial. The techs were extra gentle. The angles were steeper. My skin had the vividness of fresh paint and the temperament to match. People asked if I would ring the bell. I said maybe. The ritual lands differently in different bodies. For me the daily rite had been modest: arrive, lie still, breathe, leave.

On the final morning—late January 2024—the tech helped me slip the robe from my shoulders, and I smiled at the ceiling tile with the painted blue sky because it had been kind. When it was over, I rang the bell. Not dainty. Bar-close loud. You don't have to go home, but you can't stay here. The sound lodged somewhere between sternum and memory. The Flatirons watched me walk out bare-necked in the cold, skin too raw for a coat.

Fallout (and Falling Back In)

After radiation comes the part no one plans a ceremony for: the month where your skin peels like bark, dry curls revealing new pink beneath. My chest tightened; my armpit sulked; fascia acted precious. PT returned with its benevolent coercion—coaxing motion from a body that had excellent reasons to be guarded. We worked on ribs that had locked down like bear-proof containers. We pulled space back into them so lungs could expand and shoulders could abduct and rotate without negotiation.

Then came the slow-motion consequences. About a month after radiation ended, my right implant started to feel... purposeful. Over the next six months that capsule tightened bit by bit, until one morning I realized I had a perky, tight, incontrovertible B-cup and, on the other side, a more natural C-cup doing its ski-slope thing. I could laugh about it when I wasn't crying in the closet. Prosthetics helped, until they didn't—annoying little silicone negotiations I resented having to manage. Eventually surgery scraped out scar tissue—carefully, methodically. It treated the pain. The lopsidedness lingered until a future surgery.

Lymphedema settled in, months after the last zap. My right upper arm learned to hold fluid, confused by missing nodes and complicated scarring, a low tide that wouldn't drain. We added compression sleeves to the spreadsheet. My throat settled into a new normal—permanently raspy after two minutes of cheering, seductively quiet in theaters whether I meant to be or not. My thyroid shriveled into an ultrasound rumor that took determined probing to locate, and my Hashimoto's flared in response—swinging me between hypo and hyper while we adjusted synthetic hormones like a radio dial that refuses to land on the song.

If chemo was thunder—loud, obvious, rearranging the furniture—radiation was the weather it left behind: the daily, disciplined rain that changes the landscape and convinces you it's just being weather.

Between clinic and home, I tried to keep my life small and sturdy. Coffee stayed domestic—I could dictate temperature, foam, kindness. Scented foot cream, banned during chemo, came back like a contraband joy. Small wins. Scott became the keeper of my back, smoothing in what I couldn't reach, reading my skin with his palms. I learned the looseness of shirts that didn't make me swear and avoided fabrics with coarse opinions.

Two weeks after radiation ended, oral chemo with Xeloda began. If radiation was a machine's language, Xeloda was constitutional. It lived in a weekly organizer in the kitchen, next to the coffee beans, asking for water and patience. Ordinary, on purpose. It made me tired. It made me constipated. No plot twist there—just a plod.

And then: the email. Mid-February, my last undergraduate semester, my inbox flashing with the subject line that rearranged the furniture I thought chemo had already moved. I'd been accepted to grad school. I remember the way the light hit the kitchen table as I read it twice to be sure. Then I said Scott's name the way you say a spell. We didn't do a dance; we did something smaller and better. We breathed at the same time. Work would be hard while immunocompromised, on Xeloda, with a couple of fall surgeries on the calendar. School was a way to aim my life at a future I could believe in without promising more than a semester at a time.

What Quiet Taught Me

Quiet taught me to measure days by practice, not performance. To trust the small, boring rituals: park, breathe, align, thank, lotion, music, home. To name the weather—inside and out—without making it scenery or fate. To let help in where I couldn't reach. To understand that steady doesn't mean easy; it means I kept showing up for a machine that hummed light through me on purpose.

Radiation burned deep; uncertainty lives deeper. When the appointments stopped, the mind got loud; but the house still stood, and my life kept knocking. I had a bell tone lodged in my ribs, a chest that knew new weather, and a calendar that said keep going. I kept going.

People ask, "How was radiation?" I say "steady," and then I add the truth that doesn't fit on a clipboard: it was winter with a warm chest, a season where the brightest thing in the room was also the thing that hurt me—and helped me most. It was nipples under a T-shirt at Christmas and saying no to a fireplace for a season. It was Scott's hands and alt-rock at 8:12 a.m. Weather you learned to name, then outlast. It was a quiet burn that didn't need applause to be real.

After the bell came pills. After the pills came plans. Not in pen—never again in pen—but in confident pencil, dark enough to see, light enough to change. And when I looked west from the deck in the mornings, the mountains were still there. Beautiful. Stoic. Iconic. Not telling me anything I didn't already know, and somehow saying, "Keep going."

PART II

The Body in Revolt

Popping My Pit and Other Intimacies

The First Unveiling

The first time I saw my chest without bandages, I cried. Not from shock, but because everything arrived at once: relief, grief, relief, rage, relief again. I looked patchworked—swollen, bruised, crosshatched with steri-strips and purple marker. Reconstruction happened the same day as the mastectomy: one surgeon removed, the other rebuilt, direct-to-implant. Efficient on paper and in reality. In the mirror: implant edges visible, scar tissue already roping into little waves, one side riding higher. Not restored. Not returned. Reimagined—beautiful and flawed in the same breath.

Steam ghosted the mirror. The water stayed lukewarm on purpose, tracing a map I no longer recognized. Glue released in chemical sighs; Sharpie halos blurred. When I stepped out of the shower, air hit my chest, and I felt nothing where everything should be. My brain kept sending a courier with a message and finding no office at that address. Scott and I made Frankenstein jokes. We laughed enough to keep moving.

Borrowed Nervous System

Before, intimacy had lyrics—seduction, timing, mood lighting. After, it was jazz: improvised, honest, sometimes off-key. I don't do still. But there I was, stitched and taped, learning a different kind of strength—the kind that lets someone else hold you steady while your nervous system relearns "safe." Scott didn't just change the dressings; he kept time so my breath could find the downbeat. Co-regulator isn't romantic language, but it's the closest word for what saved me. When I startled from a lightning-bolt nerve zap, he exhaled for both of us until my body remembered how.

Pro Tips from the Pit

Drains turned me into a reluctant engineer. Two tubes exited my sides after the mastectomy, one after the node dissection—grenade bulbs collecting rust-colored tea that proved healing is messy. I logged output twice a day like a shift supervisor. My arms hugged close; I walked like a T-rex to avoid snagging a tube on the tyranny of doorknobs. I skipped opioids; the side effects cost more than the pain. Scott learned how to strip the drains, and then buckled my seatbelt, zipped my hoodie, and held my water bottle like it was a relay baton. There is no way to be dignified when your body is a plumbing project.

Ghost Map, New Wiring

A mastectomy is an amputation; the body's map gets redrawn without approval. My nervous system didn't get the update. Sensation turned into bad GPS—"Recalculating…"—pinging exits that no longer exist. A phantom itch on a breast that isn't there. Electrified assaults down my tricep because a sacrificed nerve kept sending signals to an endpoint that was gone. One minute I'd reach for a cabinet; the next, a jolt ricocheted to my elbow. Not drama—misfired wiring.

Barometric (But Make It Bodily)

Implants don't have circulation. Even when I'm sweating, my chest keeps its own atmosphere—immune to the laws of thermodynamics. Try explaining that at a barbecue. The disconnect—cold, numb, no feedback—makes the chest feel attached more than integrated. As if old copper wiring was ripped out and replaced with Bluetooth, the signal drops at random. Because there's no warning system, certain equipment is permanently retired: underwire bras (too risky), heating pads (burn hazard), ice packs (same). From clavicle to rib: diplomatic zone—neutral, unresponsive, annoyingly efficient. It's absurd and it's real; both can be true before breakfast.

A Little Off the Thigh, a Little On the Top

Let's define fat grafting. The name sounds spa-adjacent; the process is… not. It's liposuction—yes, actual lipo—from the thighs and hips (in my case), then processing that fat so only the "good stuff" remains and reinjecting it into the chest using a constellation of tiny syringes.

The "processing" step deserves its own sitcom. They essentially purify your fat—as if it's a cold-pressed extra-virgin you—from slurry to silky. Every OR has a method: strainers, filters, centrifuges. Imagine your cells riding a salad spinner of destiny until they're deemed artisanal enough to relocate. The surgeon uses dozens of micro-injections to thread that purified fat over the implant and under thin skin, sculpting volume where tissue is scarce.

Why do it? Because my remaining tissue was so thin I was basically translucent; the implant edges showed like a spoiler alert. I needed extra fat for coverage, cushioning, and to make the mirror less of a jump scare.

Recovery hurt like a motherf—well, like liposuction. Indigo flooded my thighs and hips, mellowing to mustard and old-avocado green. Compression garments vacuum-sealed everything from waist to knee. Sitting down was choreography; standing up needed a pep talk; stairs required a vulnerability TED Talk. The chest, most insensate, behaved like the subdued tenant in a noisy building. Over months, half the grafted fat reabsorbed (your body edits its own edits). What stayed softened the edges, blurred the outlines, made tops less argumentative. Detail work. A final draft, not an original. Worth it.

CSI: Armpit

The seroma was less poetic and more… sprinkler. After the lymph drain came out, a pocket of fluid set up camp in my armpit. Before the incision fully sealed, pale yellow seeped out between stitches. At the clinic, my surgeon reopened a corner, massaged out a spray of berry-colored clots, then a ribbon of lymph. Equal parts fascinating and disgusting. At home I tried daily self-massage; oddly satisfying until angle and pressure defeated me. Enter Scott: pit-popping partner. We counted clots like a deranged game show. "Four tonight." "Only two? Progress." One triumphant night—nothing. Victory arrived. Then a warm shower melted the scab, and my armpit became a rogue lawn sprinkler, an indecent arc that hit the tile with cheerful incivility. I clamped instinctively and yelled for gauze. Pop, drain, dry, repeat—for a week—until the pocket surrendered and the skin sealed. Life throws this at you and keeps walking. You're left with supplies, humor, and someone willing to do a job you can't put on a chore chart.

Wardrobe War Room

Clothes, meanwhile, became anthropology. Scars multiplied: the port site reopened and healed a deeper purple; a blunt incision crossed my chest; axillary scars curled into my pit. Tank tops turned into show-and-tell. My breasts were indisputably lopsided now—the right side tightened and rode high while the left kept its natural hang. Horizontal stripes were not invited; they underlined the difference with graphic enthusiasm.

Lymphedema puffed my upper right arm. Sleeves became tourniquets. Fabric bulged at the hem. Sizing up wasn't fashion; it was blood flow, complicated by the compression sleeve that became my new accessory. Shopping shifted from expression to strategy—comfort, concealment, control—until I could recognize myself again. On good days I let the lines show and called them stoicism. On other days I wore a cardigan and chose softness over explanation. I don't dress to hide; I dress to decide. Both were honest.

The Last Straw (Was an Eyelash)

Hair told its own story. Eyelashes were the last straw. You can accessorize a head; you can't fake fringe. Wind stung, dust won. I stashed drops in every bag like a dehydrated squirrel. Regrowth ghosted me—stubs, gone; stubs, gone—until one day they stayed. Hair came back darker, coarser, skeptical. Eyebrows phoned it in for months. My face remembered me slowly, the way a familiar room looks wrong after someone moves the furniture two inches to the left.

Perks threaded through the mess: I could get out the door fast. No hair. No mascara. A limited wardrobe—the braless relief of numb skin that didn't argue with elastic. Months went by before I needed to shave. Small efficiencies inside big negotiations.

House Rules (Post-Op Edition)

1. If the garment has opinions (seam, underwire, aggressive lace), it's uninvited.
2. If it requires explanation to a stranger in the produce section, we're saving it for later.
3. If it swells, support it; if it leaks, label it; if it zaps, swear, then breathe.
4. Accessibility beats aesthetics, unless aesthetics brings snacks.
5. Laugh when possible. Apply lotion when not.

FAQ for Well-Meaning Humans

Q: Does it hurt?
A: Not on a schedule. Pain shows up when it wants and leaves when it's done.

Q: Can you feel anything?
A: Yes. Just not where you'd assume.

Q: Do they feel real? Can I feel them?
A: To me: sometimes. To you: yes, they feel real. If I want

> you to touch me, I'll tell you. Consent isn't cancer-dependent.
>
> **Q:** How can I help?
> **A:** Ask what today's rules are. They change less than you'd think and more than I'd like.

People ask how I feel. The longer version lives in the overlap of numb and tender, fine and flattened, functional and furious. It lives in the jolt that still surprises me, and the nightly check for swelling. In the mirror, in the missing, in the new shape of ordinary.

Some days I could live in my body; some days I couldn't. I learned to choose who gets access to the archive. Strangers don't get the footnotes; they get "I'm okay." The people who've earned it get the appendix: the cold chest in a hot room, the lawn-sprinkler pit, the sleeves that prosecute circumference, the way a body can be both mine and bewildering.

The Art of Ordinary Rescue

What saved me was smaller than anyone imagines: towels warmed in the dryer; a lanyard and safety pins so I could shower on my own; soft tees pre-vetted for seam betrayal; the flicker of an unscented candle. The day had a protocol: count breaths, swap bandages, laugh at the wrong moment on purpose. Ordinary. Somehow sublime.

I wish I could say I became braver. What I became was more honest—about the body I live in and the people who live alongside it. Courage wasn't grand; it was verb-level: strip, clean, tape, lift, warm, hold. Scott kept coming with gauze and steadiness. I kept coming with a body that needed both.

Together we practiced ordinary rescue —unromantic, relentless, real.

I am not restored. I am reimagined.

The wins are small and real: a shirt that doesn't swear at my scars; an armhole that forgives; a partner who knows where the supplies live. I got a self I can live in—stitched, monitored, revised. And then I catch myself in the bathroom mirror—steam thinning, lines settling—I see it: not a before or an after, but a woman in mid-translation, learning the language of a body remade. I meet her eyes. I nod like we're in on the same joke.

Then I get on with it.

I Lost My Boobs, Hair, and Ovaries... But Not Myself

ALTERED: The Ghosts in the Mirror

Cancer took a lot. My breasts. My ovaries. My hair. My sense of autonomy. But what it didn't take was the self beneath all that—my core, my grit, my me.

I once burst into tears while brushing my teeth. Not theatrical, just an overflow. Patchy hair, puffy eyes, bruised skin. A stranger in my sweatshirt stared back. I thought reclaiming would feel like arrival. It felt like unraveling. Turns out, unraveling is its own kind of becoming.

Top 10 Things Cancer Stole From Me

1. Boobs. Front and center. Gone. They look like breasts but feel like stand-ins.
2. Hair. Shaving it felt like agency; regrowth felt like betrayal—like the world wanted me to pretend nothing happened.
3. Ovaries—and my last natural hormones. Surgically evicted. Welcome to medical menopause: hot flashes

mood swings, bone aches, insomnia—the Hellfire & Hormones starter kit.

4. Naïve Faith in My Body. I thought we were teammates. Then it turned on me from the inside. Now we're on a fragile truce.
5. Sleep. Rest became folklore. Sleep deprivation blurs grief and sharpens anxiety.
6. Mirror Confidence. The version I recognized vanished. Mangy hair, faded lashes, mottled skin. A liminal face.
7. Social Energy. I now budget life. Some days the entire allowance disappears on brushing my teeth.
8. Long-Term Plans. The future comes with an asterisk. Hope, with a side of hesitation.
9. Old Femininity Rules. Destabilizing at first; ultimately liberating.
10. Pretending I'm Fine. Filter: gone. I don't small-talk weather; I lunch-talk grief and nipple reconstruction. Sorry not sorry.

Loss took inventory. Endurance kept the books.

I felt misread—quiet read as cold, honesty as hostility. Chemo burned my bandwidth for performance. I stopped pretending. A quick grocery run proved how exposed I was: scarf as armor, eyes on me, pity (some real, some imagined). I felt like shopping naked—wearing only pink-ribbon pasties and unspoken grief.

Public grief is performance. Private grief is a roommate.

After midnight, courage has a different weight. The house asleep, the refrigerator hums like a distant ocean and I lie on my back and count stitches I can't see anymore, replaying conversations I wish I'd had—with doctors, with friends, with myself. Grief arrives in pajamas and makeup-free; she sits on the edge of the bed and refuses small talk. I don't try to outthink her. I make room. I name what hurts out loud—whispered, so I don't wake anyone: fear of recurrence, anger at randomness, tenderness for the version of me who still hoped chemo would be smooth sailing. Sometimes I cry; sometimes I just listen. When the wave passes, I write one sentence on a sticky note: You are still here. I stick it to the nightstand, turn off the lamp, and let the dark be kind. By morning, I don't feel victorious. I feel honest. That's enough to stand up.

INTACT: The Ember Still Burning

Even when the mirror returned a stranger, an ember of personhood glowed—stubborn, background uninterrupted. If I could crack a pit-popping joke or consider bedazzling my compression sleeve, I hadn't vanished. Absurdity survived: drains, blue pee, "axillary dissection" sounding like a punk band.

What makes me a woman now? Estrogen or endurance? Ovaries or sovereignty? Some days: spiritual. Other days: "Hell if I know." Either way, the center held.

Top 7 Things Cancer Couldn't Take

1. My Voice. I still name what others prefer glossed. Truth-telling as creative resistance.
2. My People. Soup, playlists, dark humor. They didn't need me inspirational; they needed me real.
3. My Grit. Not pinkwashed perseverance—just showing up for scan #19 and texting back five days later, emoji included.
4. My Humor. Armor and release.

5. My Mind. Chemo fogged logistics, not curiosity. Metaphor sharp. Sarcasm sharp. Social commentary sharp.
6. My Right to Rage. Systems are broken. Rage is a focusing lens, not a flaw.
7. My Compassion. Wider now—for others and for myself.

Being intact isn't the same as belonging to your body. That took practice.

RECLAIMED: Living in the Afterbody

I didn't bounce back. I crawled out—bruised, limping, unsure how to fly. Healing wasn't a triumph; it was amnesty. The afterbody remembers the scar tissue and nerve maps, numb patches and surprise aches. Reclaiming happened in fragments: clothes that felt like me again, a calendar that wasn't built around blood draws, walking with scars visible and my head up.

The first time I wore a V-neck in public, my port scar showing, I braced. Instead, I felt... real. Not flaunting trauma—refusing to bury it. This is the body I live in now. Not untouched, but undeniably mine. Femininity returned different—a new rhythm. Not heels and lipstick, but boundaries and staying soft without being small.

Habits changed. Getting dressed became a safety check: gentleness over scars, sleeves that support swelling, necklines that don't tug at sensitive skin. Bras turned political: underwire out, soft cups in, then—for a while—no bra at all. Rebellion and relief. Showering became navigation, not autopilot—gentle movement around surgical sites and numb patches. Hair care became deliberate: chemo fuzz shampoo, "chemo curls = it'll grow back better" mantras, and the day I stopped reaching for a ponytail holder.

Food shifted, too. Chemo betrayed my taste buds. Prosecco and charcuterie became soda water and chocolate chip tahini cake. Still celebration—just reframed.

But the reclaiming didn't stop at the front door. I had to reclaim the clinic, too.

Time moves in scan cycles. I don't do lucky socks. I do strategy. I leave ten minutes early because hospital parking is a morality play. I pack ginger chews, moisturizer for the tape rash, and a pen for consent forms that never remember my middle initial. I bring the playlist that keeps my heart rate under 80—soulful, steady, no surprise cymbals. I wear short sleeves, so the phlebotomist at least has a fighting chance. We usually take four stabs to hit pay dirt; halfway through, he jokes that even my veins are fatigued. Sometimes they vanish mid-draw like they found a trapdoor. We start again.

Post-scan, my treat is deliberately ordinary: a grocery store bouquet and a chocolate–peanut butter–banana protein shake. If results day is a cliff, ritual is my railing. When the portal dings, I text: "Opening now. Please love me even if I'm feral." Survival used to mean white-knuckling the unknown. Now it means building a small, repeatable kindness around it.

The first time I stepped into a river after surgery, the water negotiated with my scars before it greeted me—every seam, every numb peninsula. Temperature announced itself in gradients my nerves no longer map. I moved slowly, an accord between fear and muscle memory. Waist-deep, I realized my body had remembered something I'd forgotten: float. Not lightness—buoyancy as physics, proof I could be held. I cried as

I paddled. I felt strong in a new key—less violin, more cello. Deeper, resonant, mine.

I started wanting things again; not just to get through, but to live. To plan trips without calculating clot risk. To laugh so hard I forget my medication list. To forgive on purpose, not to smooth things over but to align with my values. To honor my ghosts without being governed by them. Practice turned into pattern. Pattern turned into direction.

Top 10 Things I've Reclaimed

1. My Right to Exist As I Am. No apologies. No hiding. Enough now, not later.
2. My Voice in the Exam Room. I ask, I push, I say no. Care should honor me.
3. My Body, As It Is. New geography, same tenant. I respect it.
4. My Energy. Different? Yes. Depleted? Sometimes. Mine to spend where it matters most.
5. My Mind. Fog lingers, and clarity comes in the form of perspective, persistence, presence.
6. My Boundaries. Peace is sacred. I protect it.
7. My Beauty. Rooted in how I show up, not how I look.
8. My Humor. Still dark. Still weird. Still barbed. It survived everything.
9. My Wisdom. Hard-earned. Bone deep.
10. My Wholeness. I lost parts, not myself.

I used to live in conflict with my scars—they told a story I didn't choose. Then I tried naming them. Names that told my story. The crescent under my arm became Switchback. The faded square where my port lived became Confluence. The tightest line across my chest—Crux. Once things had names, they stopped being foreign. I could talk to them: "What the... Crux?!" They were places I've been. I stopped bracing for pity and started asking for what I needed: a slower hug, a softer shirt, five minutes to breathe. Naming wasn't glamour. It was grammar. It let me make sentences again.

Afterbody Field Guide (Pocket Edition)

Uniform: Soft seams, easy exits, pockets for snacks and courage.

Hydration: Water tastes better out of a bottle covered in stickers. This is science* (*feelings).

Movement: Ten minutes counts. So does dancing while the coffee brews.

Social: Two-hour cap on events. Leave while you still like people.

Medical Admin: Calendar = external brain. Portal messages = haikus of assertiveness.

Joy: Schedule it. If you don't, something loud will take its place.

Grief: Comes uninvited. Set a chair. Don't let it drive.

There's a bench by the river where I practice doing nothing on purpose. I used to think healing would feel like fireworks; lately it feels like catching sunlight on my knees. I watch a dog fail spectacularly at fetching a stick and congratulate him anyway. I peel an orange, mindfully. I eavesdrop on a toddler narrating the universe: rock, bird, sky, mine. The ache in my ribs makes its small announcement; I put a hand there and nod back. A cyclist clatters past and the world continues, shockingly, without my permission.

For a long time, I mistook endurance for denial. Now I understand it as attention. When the river runs high, it is loud and insistent. When it is low, I can see the sculpted stones. Both are the river. Both are true. On the walk home I rehearse a sentence I used to be afraid to say out loud: I love this life, exactly as it is, even when it hurts. The grief isn't gone. It's just not the only voice in the room.

Living in the afterbody means living with paradox: I am softer, and stronger. I am scarred, and radiant. I am altered, and intact. I am broken open, and somehow whole.

Living Forward: My North Stars

No more resolutions. I've written enough survival plans. I need solid footholds to keep me secure in the ever-shifting terrain of survivorship.

Mind: Clarity isn't control; it's persistence. I choose myself, even when the path is obscured.

Body: Altered, aching, astonishing. I move with curiosity, not critique. I honor it with care and awe, treating it as an ally, not an adversary.

Voice: I advocate for myself—in clinics, in conversation, in the mirror. I ask, I push, I say no. Care should honor me.

Energy: The sacred currency. I spend it wisely, save it guilt-free, and give only where it nourishes. I listen to my body's cues. Rest counts.

Spirit: The unuttered throughline. I celebrate progress—especially when it's slow.

Self: Evolved. Someone I trust. I live authentically and unapologetically: messy, defiant, funny, scarred, and bone-deep wise.

I did not walk through fire to be restored to who I was. That version of me is gone—and that's not a loss; it's a becoming.

I am not what the fire spared. I am what the fire forged.

Invisibility, Tokenism, Inspirational

The first support group I joined was an online grid of kind strangers and a silence I could feel in my ribs. Someone read a devotional. Someone else held up a gratitude journal. I stared at my own square—bald, gray shirt, eyes like low tide—and tried to swallow a feeling that didn't fit the script. When it was my turn, I said, "Hi, I'm Jill," and then nothing. The room nodded for me anyway.

I logged off and sighed, not because anyone was cruel, but because I could not find myself inside their version of hope.

The Myth of the Inspirational Survivor

The sanitized story is the one that wins hearts. It's where the survivor finds clarity and appreciation and walks into the sunset with a new lease on life. Bonus points if she looks good bald and talks about how cancer made her stronger.

The dominant narrative—the undefeated survivor who radiates gratitude—gets reinforced everywhere. In Hallmark cards, pink-ribbon campaigns, feel-good news clips, and the "you got this" hashtags peppered across social media. Cancer, in these depictions, is less a disease and more a spiritual boot camp designed to produce better humans.

I never wanted to star in that story. I don't even understand it—if it exists at all.

At first, I kept quiet on Instagram. No shaved-head selfies. No marathon-style treatment countdowns. No curated images of bravery through tears. I kept the circle small—not because I was ashamed, but because I didn't want to perform for an algorithm, to turn my illness into content. I didn't want "likes" accumulating on my suffering like confetti at a pity party. I wasn't interested in collecting inspirational points for surviving something I never asked to endure.

Eventually, I did post something—once I had words that held both the pain and the complexity. I shared the picture carousel: some with hair, some with scarves, and some bald. I wrote honestly:

> One year today, a radiologist sat next to me explaining that my diagnostic mammogram looked suspicious. Numerous imaging studies and two biopsies later, breast cancer was confirmed. I was devastated. Over the past year, cancer has been consuming, enlightening, surprising, and humbling. In 7 months, I underwent a bilateral mastectomy with direct-to-implant reconstruction surgery, followed by 4 rounds of chemo, and breast revision surgery.
>
> Four weeks later, a routine blood test revealed abnormally high tumor markers. Numerous imaging studies and two biopsies later, cancer recurrence was confirmed. Surgery

> to remove malignant lymph nodes revealed the disease was more extensive than originally thought and to complicate things, two different types of breast cancer were present—both of which were different from the first.
>
> Today I started the first of twelve rounds of chemo, which will be followed by six and a half weeks of daily radiation. I'm grateful for many things—my cancer being caught early TWICE, strong love and support from my tribe, and an amazing care team that appreciates my tenacity and use of the F word. Friends—check some tits—yours or someone else's (with consent, of course!).

Even then, it felt complicated. The comments came in—many of them tender and real. But the likes from people I didn't know? That felt strange, voyeuristic even. As if my illness had suddenly made me more visible—but only in the ways that fit their expectations. I wasn't looking for a spotlight. I was just trying to live as openly and honestly as I could.

There's a cultural script waiting for us the moment we're diagnosed. It's optimistic, relentless, and oddly performative. You've seen it: the glowing Instagram photo, bald head kissed by sunlight, captioned with something like "Cancer picked the wrong girl" or "Thriving through the storm." These stories are shared widely, celebrated publicly. They're a balm to the well-meaning. Proof, supposedly, that attitude is everything.

But they double as traps—ones lined with sequins and slogans. Here's what that myth constructs:

> **Performance pressure:** Be brave, be grateful, be photogenic.
> **Self-blame:** If you're not thriving, you must be doing survivorship wrong.
> **Erasure:** Difference gets cropped out—age, race, class, queerness, fertility, access.

In the early days of my diagnosis, I clung to those stories like life rafts. I wanted to believe them. I needed to believe that with the right mindset, I could muscle my way through this thing and come out looking fabulous and full of perspective. That maybe cancer wouldn't interrupt my life so much as lightly brush against it. That maybe I could just... do it better. Cleaner.

I remember reading a post on a breast cancer forum from a woman who fit the super-survivor mold so well it made my teeth hurt. She proudly shared that her mastectomy hadn't interrupted her work—she missed only a couple of days and returned full-time, no big deal. I read it while recovering from my mastectomy, having just made the gut-wrenching decision to withdraw from my respiratory therapy program.

I was propped up on pillows, drained—literally and figuratively—trying to manage pain, grief, and tubing stitched into my sides. Her words felt like a slap wrapped in a smile. That's what I wanted: minimal disruption. But that wasn't my reality. Reading her life as the standard bruised something in me I didn't have words for yet.

The lesson I learned over and over: every case of breast cancer is different. Every survivor walks a different path. There is no standard. There is only your body, your life, your timing.

After losing my hair to chemo, I became obsessed with regrowth timelines. I stumbled across a blog where a woman documented her hair journey in photos: one month, two months, six, ten, fifteen. The final photo showed her in her kitchen, beaming, blonde hair cascading past her shoulders and down her back. It was beautiful. She was beautiful. My heart lifted—proof that recovery could be quick. I wouldn't have to live in scarves or hats for long.

But just as I was closing the tab, I noticed a tiny asterisk at the bottom of the post: hair extensions used.

I felt the floor drop out. Why hadn't she disclosed this up front? In a moment of vulnerability, I believed I was looking at what was possible when, in fact, I was looking at something enhanced, polished, edited.

That's the thing about the inspirational survivor myth—it glosses over the pain, the complications, the accommodations, the long shadows that follow treatment. It reduces survival to a personal triumph narrative, when in reality, survival is often a negotiated truce between your body, your spirit, and the systems meant to care for you.

We crave these stories because they promise certainty. A roadmap. Hope that looks good in a selfie. And sometimes they do help. Sometimes we need to see the light at the end of someone else's tunnel. But when they become the only stories we hear—or worse, the stories we feel expected to live up to—they start to erase the complexity of truth. They flatten the jaggedness of survivorship into something digestible, photogenic, and misleading.

I sought out those stories because I was scared. I wanted something to orient myself. But I've since learned that there is strength in showing the un-Instagrammable moments too—in the tears behind the bathroom door, the unfinished to-do list, the shaved head that doesn't feel empowering at all. We need more than curated victories. We need the whole story.

Invisibility and Tokenism in Cancer Culture

Late one night, early in my diagnosis, I sat in bed scrolling through cancer forums. The house was quiet except for the occasional faraway train whistle and the soft exhale of Scott asleep beside me. I wasn't just looking for another woman with ER/PR+ disease. I was searching for someone whose life looked like mine. Someone with a loving irreverent partner. Someone fluid in their sexuality. The parent of queer kids. Living in a neighborhood where everyone's not the same shade. Someone who knew their way around irony and intimacy and who didn't find comfort in pink boxing gloves or the phrase "you got this."

But that's not who I found.

Mostly, I saw white, cis women in their sixties and seventies. Hair silvering or tucked under elaborate scarves. Tastefully dressed. Maybe a tiny gold cross resting against a delicate clavicle. They made cancer look… refined. As if the whole thing could be survived with grace, matching jewelry, and a side of cucumber water.

I wasn't looking for elegance. I was looking for truth.

I didn't want an 80-year-old stranger assuring me that she still had an active sex life. I didn't want advice that read like it was sponsored by a luxury retreat center. I wasn't looking for anonymous complaints without context. I wanted someone thoughtful, maybe even skeptical. Someone who could sit inside contradiction. Who understood both the science and the soul of it.

The longer I scrolled, the colder the screen felt. Insights were rare—a phrase to bring up at my next oncology appointment, a therapy I hadn't heard of yet—but mostly, those forums felt shallow or radioactive. And I didn't have the capacity to absorb everyone else's trauma when I was barely holding my own.

Queerness doesn't vanish with a cancer diagnosis. Complexity doesn't evaporate under the hospital gown. If anything, illness made me more defiant about being fully myself. It didn't simplify me—it deepened me. Mother. Partner. Artist. Student. Survivor. Advocate. Skeptic. All of it mattered. And I wasn't going to peel off those layers just to make someone else more comfortable with my story.

That night, scrolling and not finding myself, I began to understand the difference between inclusion and belonging. Representation wasn't just about images. It was about access to community, to care, to the basic dignity of being seen. Inclusion is being let in the room; belonging is being able to exhale there.

Every now and then, you'll spot a Black or Brown face in a cancer brochure. But they're rare—like someone was photoshopped in at the last minute to check a box. You have to search even harder to find a queer face. Men, though they do get breast cancer, are almost entirely invisible. And young women, despite the rising numbers? Gone. As absent as the information about fertility, which too often is either buried, inaccessible, or completely ignored.

Public narratives, especially during October, lean heavily on the pink ribbon parade. Walks and runs and rallies, all filled with smiling faces and slogans about strength. Survivors wear branded buttons and sashes like party favors—arms pumped skyward in a show of triumph. The merch is everywhere. Pink yogurt lids. Pink drill bits. Pink NFL cleats. Breast cancer awareness, brought to you by the same people who gave us cheese-stuffed crusts.

When I first really saw these campaigns, I was on the couch, too weak to sit upright. Chemo had flattened me. My immune system bottomed out. I couldn't walk around the block let alone join a crowd of thousands. Those posters didn't inspire me. They felt like propaganda. They didn't speak to risk factors or reproductive decisions or access to quality care. They didn't name systemic racism, medical mistrust, or what it's like to be dismissed by your provider because you don't look like the "typical" breast cancer patient.

Those pink ribbons were cute, curated, commercial. I felt alienated from the movement supposedly built for me. Tokenism pretends to be inclusion. But it just puts difference behind glass—admired, contained, untouched.

And yet, two years after my first diagnosis, I found myself at a breast cancer fundraiser. My son's fraternity had a team registered in an organized 5k walk, and Scott and I flew to Iowa to join him. I didn't know what to expect—mostly, I braced for discomfort.

But the sea of people, the sheer magnitude of it, caught me off guard. I teared up more than once walking through that crowd, my son's fraternity letters stretched across my back. Not because it was pink and cheerful, but because it was messy. Real. Sweaty and awkward and unfiltered. This time, it wasn't pink-washed strength. It was community. And I belonged to it.

As we walked, I noticed the backs of others' t-shirts. The slogans, not just the corporate ones—Team General Mills, matching socks and all—but the homemade ones. Tina's Tribe. My Boobs Tried to Kill Me. Thanks for the Mammories. Boobs: They Need Support. Hope Unleashes Your Superpower. In Memory of Aunt Helen. Each shirt told a story. Some made me laugh out loud. Some made me pause. Some made me ache.

It was dark humor, lightness, grief, grit, hope, corporate branding, friendship bracelets, survivors with bald heads and crooked smiles, family members holding signs, toddlers in tutus. All the things. As diverse and complex as cancer itself.

Afterward, I realized something I hadn't let myself admit before: as frustrating as the pink campaigns can be, all those yogurt lids and NFL cleats do serve a purpose. They open the door. They start conversations. They normalize talking about breasts—and about what happens when our bodies betray us. Sometimes, that's enough to spark a question, a memory, a mammogram, a moment of connection.

It doesn't excuse the oversimplification. But it reminds me that even flawed visibility can be a first step. And sometimes, the first step is enough to carry someone toward their own story. Their own beginning.

The Side Effects No One Talks About

Some side effects come with leaflets. Others come with shame.

Chemo brain showed up early. I once stood in the kitchen holding a bag of coffee beans, staring at the espresso machine like it was alien technology. I couldn't remember the next step. My brain—once sharp and efficient—turned foggy and unreliable. Words slipped away mid-sentence. I'd start a thought and abandon it without meaning to. I felt dumb in a way I couldn't talk myself out of. I lost confidence mid-conversation, unable to recall the word for "zip-line" or how to explain what day it was.

Constipation was next level. Not just inconvenient—crippling. There were days I couldn't stand up straight. I became fiercely loyal to MiraLAX. I should have bought stock. Or at least gotten a loyalty card. I kept a special bottle of juice in the fridge with my name on it—not because I loved it, but because it was laced with laxatives and I couldn't risk anyone else drinking it. "Do not touch—this will ruin your day," I wanted to write on the label.

Then there were the invisible things. The ones no one warned me about. The kind that don't get hashtags or ribbon colors.

Neuropathy that made buttoning a shirt a test of patience. Nerve pain that left phantom echoes in the space where my breasts used to be. Medical menopause handed to me without ceremony. Grief I didn't know how to name. PTSD woven into routine scans and waiting rooms. Anxiety that hid in the corners even when I was surrounded by love.

There is a cost to surviving that no one prepares you for. The body logs it. The mind audits it. And then, just when you think you've made it through the worst of it—when the hair starts growing back, the appointments are slightly more spaced out—you're expected to rejoin the world.

For the record: I eventually made the espresso. And then, because I'm apparently incapable of accepting mystery, I started calculating what I did to earn the rest.

The Loneliness Between

I did what so many of us do: I turned inward and hunted for the root cause like it was a puzzle I'd failed to solve. I blamed myself. Thoroughly. I replayed every happy hour I'd ever had. I wondered if the chemicals I used to clean my counters, the stress I carried for years, or the hormones in my birth control had tipped the scales. The air I breathed, the city I lived in, the plastics I used?

I turned my life into a case study in personal failure. As if I had invited cancer in and let it make itself at home. I needed a way out of that spiral of self-blame.

Which brought me back to the grid of faces on my laptop screen. At that first cancer support group—the one with the devotionals and gratitude journals—I felt more alone on Zoom than I ever did on my own shower floor. Most of the women were older, straight, and married. They spoke tenderly of husbands who shaved their heads in solidarity or neighbors who brought them soup in bed. Heads nodding, trying to match their rhythm, I felt myself slipping out of sync.

I didn't see myself there, not as someone still processing the injustice of it all. I wasn't looking for someone to tell me it would be okay. I was looking for someone to say, This is hard. And weird. And sometimes awful. And yes, it's okay to be angry.

You can be surrounded by kind people and still feel soul-lonely—especially if you're queer, a person of color, child-free, young, or just complicated in ways that the standard doesn't account for. The spaces meant for "healing" can sometimes deepen the ache.

There's a kind of dislocation that comes after surviving: Not sick enough to stay. Not well enough to belong.

The support groups feel too raw. The book clubs feel too trivial. The people who were your people feel like ghosts. Or worse, mirrors. You want connection, not pity. You want to be understood, not handled. So where do you go?

I started sorting spaces the way a triage nurse sorts symptoms:

Performance spaces—high polish, low honesty.

Processing spaces—big feelings, thin facts.

Practical spaces—tips and timelines, no room for grief.

I needed a fourth: **whole spaces**—where my science brain and my sore body and my complicated life could sit together without apology.

Sometimes you rebuild community in unexpected places—laughing with a pharmacy tech who remembers your name, in yoga classes where everyone sobs during savasana and no one pretends they're fine. Sometimes you find it slowly, in the shared silence of a friend who listens when you say the hard thing.

Other times, you have to build what didn't exist. A new circle, a new language, a new permission—to be unfinished, unsure, unguarded. You learn that belonging doesn't always mean fitting in. Sometimes it means being seen as you are—scarred, scared, sacred. Sometimes it's the friend who texts after your scan, the neighbor who remembers your dog's name, the fellow survivor who gets it.

Community after cancer isn't always big. But when it's real, it's medicine. The kind without a copay or side effects—unless you count snort-laughing over perfectly inappropriate songs mid-scanxiety. Like the time a routine PET scan lit up a suspicious mass in my left butt cheek. Turned out it was just inflammation from a recent Lupron shot—but an MRI was ordered to be sure.

I called Khaylen, my breastie, and before I could spiral too far, she erupted into the hook from DJ Assault's iconic "Ass 'N Titties"—full commitment, zero warning, and not a shred of regard for my remaining dignity. I had tears rolling down my cheeks. My gut hurt from the belly laughs. Something shifted. I wasn't alone. I wasn't too much. I was just... a person with radioactive ass inflammation and a friend who speaks my love language: unhinged solidarity.

That moment reminded me that two things can be true: my body can feel like a landmine, and I can still collapse into joy with someone who refuses to let me face the blast alone. Both truths fit. Both matter. And in that ridiculous, perfect rupture, the fear loosened its grip—honest, unmistakable. That's what the right people do: they wedge a little light into the dark.

Reclamation: Rage, Honesty, and the Myth of Bravery

There was so much talk about being brave, about being chosen for a reason. About letting go and letting God. But I wasn't trying to let go—I was trying to hold on. To my identity. My curiosity. My defiance. My humor. My right to be flawed and scared and still valid.

The culture keeps auditioning me for "brave." I keep declining. Bravery, as sold, is a costume; what I needed was capacity. Rage, candor, and humor weren't just coping mechanisms—they were survival tools. Tools I sharpened in real time, when platitudes felt like poison and pink ribbons made me want to scream.

Let me tell you: nothing feels less inspiring than being constipated for days, sobbing in a bathrobe while trying to shit, wondering if your new meds are turning your digestive system into concrete.

That's not a metaphor. Just my Tuesday.

Bravery wasn't what I needed. I needed to feel what I felt. To not gaslight myself into gratitude. To allow fury and sarcasm and grief and absurdity to coexist. I didn't trust my voice at first.

But I learned to. I learned that rage could be generative. That gallows humor was a form of clarity. That telling the truth out loud could make me feel less alone—even when it made others uncomfortable.

I didn't exit stage right to applause. I stayed right here, in the grit and the light of the real.

I didn't want to be brave. I wanted to be honest. And sometimes that honesty looked like rage. Sometimes it looked like silence. Sometimes it looked like tears. Sometimes it looked like talking about identity while high on Ativan. I didn't become a shinier version of myself. I didn't transform. What happened was reclamation. What happened was survival. What happened was the unavoidable collision with someone I was becoming.

Healing wasn't graceful. It was therapy. It was art. It was telling the truth without sanding off the edges.

And maybe that's the real story—not transformation into someone new, but the fierce reckoning with the parts of me I refused to abandon. The parts that demanded more room. More voice. More truth.

Cancer sure as hell didn't make me inspirational. It made me particular. It made me allergic to performance and devoted to the unedited. Most of all, it made me knowable to myself.

Built to Fail: What the System Got Exactly Right

People don't talk enough about the strategy of staying alive.

The binders. The bills. The calls. The inbox full of "This is not a bill" letters that somehow always become a bill anyway. I was fighting for my life, yes. But I was also fighting for coverage, continuity, and the right to not be charged $1,300 for a medication that cost $9 with a GoodRx coupon.

The deeper I went into treatment, the more obvious it became that the medical system wasn't failing me by accident. It was working exactly as designed—to serve those who know how to navigate it, to reward passivity, and to punish complexity.

Designed to Exhaust

At one point, I had ten doctors across multiple locations. Ten. Double digits. I was the only one who knew everything happening at any given time.

I carried my entire case history on my phone, tracked in a spreadsheet I updated like a second job. I was the one spotting potential drug interactions between specialists who'd never met, catching missing test results, noticing when a scan "fell off" the schedule like it had somewhere better to be. The system should have caught those things. It didn't.

Before cancer, I had two doctors: a primary care provider and an endocrinologist. Three years in, my medical contact list had exploded. I added a breast surgeon, a plastic surgeon, a neurologist, a radiologist, an immunologist, a podiatrist, an oncologist, and—briefly—an OB for the ovarian eviction. Plus: an acupuncturist, a physical therapist, and a rotating cast of surgical assistants.

They all did their best to communicate—faxing, messaging, occasionally sending notes via portal pigeon. But the person holding the whole story—every medication, procedure, reaction, and side effect—was me. If I forgot to mention a drug, if I didn't notice a contraindication, if I assumed "someone else" had ordered the scan—no one was going to swoop in and fix it.

At some point during cancer treatment, I stopped feeling like a patient and started feeling like the part-time administrator for a slowly imploding nonprofit—except the nonprofit was my body, and the board of directors kept voting to increase my deductible.

And here's the part that matters: I am privileged. I am white. College-educated. Middle class. Married to someone who can drive me to appointments. I speak fluent medical-ish, have reliable internet, a flexible schedule, and access to food, transportation, and a safe, comfortable home.

And still, I almost drowned.

This wasn't about one bad doctor or a single clerical error. It was about a system that depends on burnout, both from professionals and patients. It expects us to be compliant, silent, and grateful. It demands more from providers while giving them less: more boxes to click, more codes to bill, less time to think.

It's not a glitch. It's the business model.

Insurance as Obstacle Course

There's a war within the war: insurance.

We like to pretend healthcare is personal—between you and your doctor, or you and your diagnosis. It's not. There's always a third character in the room: a company deciding, in real time, whether your survival is covered.

I had to advocate for every treatment adjustment, every referral, every pain management option. I watched other patients give up—not because they didn't care, but because they didn't understand the maze or were too exhausted to keep calling. Too demoralized to fight for the care they were told they "deserved."

We're sold a script that says if you didn't get the right care, it's because you didn't try hard enough. You didn't do your research. You weren't persistent. Or worse, you didn't deserve it.

Here's what it looked like in my chart:

> **Immunotherapy drugs:** denied. My oncologist called the insurance company's medical director directly. After multiple rounds of "negotiation," they were approved—only thirty days late.
>
> **Second course of chemo:** denied. The algorithm said chemo was "medically necessary" before lymph node dissection and therefore not necessary after. Never mind that those nodes had to be removed to diagnose

the extent of my cancer in the first place. Another appeal. Another thirty-day delay.

Surgical assistants: denied for three of my toughest surgeries. Apparently the surgeon could just... grow extra hands. I filed personal appeals. Two were approved. Eleven months later, I'm still fighting the third.

Migraine meds: denied, even after trying five alternatives. Even after my neurologist explained that we needed something that wouldn't interfere with targeted therapy. Eventually approved, then denied again the next month. Same drug. Same diagnosis. New excuse.

This isn't bureaucracy. It's obstruction dressed up as process.

On paper, it's about "medical necessity." In practice, it's about who has the time, health, and rage-stamina to appeal.

Cancer's Side Hustle Is Paperwork

Cancer itself is brutal. But do you know what's actually soul-draining? Appealing the same insurance denial five times because someone behind a desk decided a surgical assistant wasn't "medically necessary," according to their interpretation, not your surgeon's.

I became frighteningly good at the appeals process. I learned the phrases that triggered internal reviews, how to escalate without getting flagged as "hostile," and could recite CPT codes like a second language. I wasn't trying to become a case manager; I just wanted to stay alive without going bankrupt.

Over the course of my treatment, I've had three different insurance policies. The second one? A bureaucratic fever dream.

They hadn't digitized their system yet. Every appeal had to be printed, completed in ink, and mailed. With a real stamp. I'm convinced they did this to weed out the weak, the tired, and anyone without access to a home printer.

I mailed in the paperwork and waited. And waited. No acknowledgment. No reply. Just the sound of time passing while someone in a windowless office misplaced my file under a box of Pinktober swag.

If the wrong field was left blank or a checkbox wasn't ticked just so, it triggered an automatic denial. Some of my appeals were rejected for formatting issues. A missing date. An "improperly aligned" signature. As if what was on the line was not a person's body, but a permission slip for a middle school field trip.

And while I had the capacity (barely) and the tenacity (also barely) to push through the system's red tape, what about the people who don't? Who are too sick. Too overwhelmed. Who don't speak the same bureaucratic dialect or have no idea where to begin appealing a decision that makes no human sense?

The emotional labor of cancer is already enough. Logistical labor should not require an unofficial degree in medical billing and advanced negotiation.

By the end of it, I had enough clinical knowledge to co-author a peer-reviewed article.

Unfortunately, I needed it to keep my insurance from ghosting me.

How to Appeal Like a Sick Person Who Doesn't Have Time for This Shit

Let's be honest: you shouldn't have to do any of this. But if you do, here are a few battle-tested tips from the trenches:

1. **Assume the first denial is automatic.** Appeal anyway. You're not crazy. They just hope you'll give up.
2. **Use their language**. Talk like a robot who's read the plan booklet. Say "medically necessary," "urgent reconsideration," and "as outlined in Section 8." Bonus points if you sound like you passed the bar.
3. **Keep receipts.** Literally. Scan and save everything. EOBs, letters, calls, appeals, timestamps, rejection notices. If spreadsheets are your love language, lean in.
4. **Escalate.** Ask for peer-to-peer reviews, medical director reviews, external reviews. Don't be afraid to name names or ask for supervisors. You're not rude. You're surviving.
5. **Phone a friend.** This is where a loved one or patient advocate is worth their weight in dark chocolate and anti-nausea meds.
6. **Note the emotional labor.** Crying on hold while explaining your diagnosis to a third-party contractor for the third time in a week? That's labor. It shouldn't be the price of care.

One Year, One Million Dollars

Behind every "miracle of modern medicine" is a billing department with a calculator and a warped sense of humor.

In my first year of treatment, the cost of staying alive totaled just over one million dollars.

Insurance covered $190,366.38. We paid $10,979.07 out of pocket—and that doesn't include mental health therapy or dry needling.

What did a million dollars buy?

Chemo. Twice. Immunotherapy. Surgeries. Ports placed, pulled, and replaced. Bone scans. Heart scans. Brain scans. Estrogen suppression. Monthly injections. Dozens of labs. Dozens of specialists. One ER visit—for the flu—because cancer torched my immune system.

It was relentless. It was necessary. It was punishing.

And the remaining $800,000-ish? Billed but never really paid. Ghost money shuffled between hospital systems and insurance algorithms. Inflated charges. Phantom costs. Fictional debt with real consequences.

Because even when no one pays the full amount, the patient still pays the price—in vigilance, in exhaustion, in the lurking fear that next time, the game won't end in your favor.

Lost in Transmission

Even the best providers are constrained by this architecture.

When I was waiting on my initial biopsy results, I got a call from my primary care physician's assistant—a woman I deeply trust, someone who'd seen me through pregnancies, autoimmune flares, a divorce, and now this. She asked gently how I was doing.

I paused. Then asked, "Are you about to tell me I have cancer?"

Silence.

Then her voice shook. The chart said the radiologist had already contacted me. I, in fact, had heard nothing. She was mortified. Apologetic. Caught in a breakdown between offices. She hadn't expected to deliver the news.

And yet, in a strange way, I was grateful. There is no perfect way to hear you have cancer, but if it had to happen, I was glad it came from someone who knew me. We cried together. She sent the pathology report immediately and called radiology to make sure follow-up happened.

Both women, the PA and the radiologist, were skilled, compassionate, and communicative.

And still, there was a snafu.

That's how this system works. Not because people don't care, but because it isn't built for continuity. It's built for throughput. For billing. For speed. For survival of the fittest.

When Your Zip Code Becomes a Diagnosis

I live within twenty miles of a cancer center. That alone makes me an outlier.

If I had been living two hours east or west—still in the same state—I might have waited three months for a PET scan. Or driven hundreds of miles for radiation. Or seen a general practitioner for a breast mass because no oncology clinic nearby had an opening.

In some zip codes, it's not about when you get care—it's about if you ever get it.

Geography becomes triage. Your address becomes a prognosis.

If you're in a rural area, you're more likely to face late diagnoses, fewer specialists, outdated equipment, and the charming suggestion to "just drive to the city." As if that's free. As if everyone has a car. As if every shift worker can miss a day—or a month.

And that's the diagnosis they never code for: time poverty.

I could make calls during business hours. I could spend forty-seven minutes on hold. I could show up, reschedule, track labs.

But what if I couldn't?

What if I were working two jobs? What if missed wages from one appointment meant an eviction notice? What if the radiation center didn't offer evening hours and the bus only ran once an hour?

The system interprets this not as lack of access, but lack of compliance. That's how it protects itself: it documents your failure instead of its design.

Debt as a Side Effect

In the U.S., surviving cancer comes with a price tag—often one you don't see clearly until your body is already wrecked and your bandwidth is gone.

For many people, cancer means debt. Full stop.

Medical debt doesn't just look like hospital bills. It shows up as maxed-out credit cards, missed rent, cashed-out retirement, delayed treatment, and GoFundMe pages passed around like collection plates. I've seen more "please share" links for medical fundraisers than baby photos. That's not community. That's policy failure wrapped in a pink ribbon.

And the burden doesn't fall evenly.

Communities of color, disabled people, LGBTQ+ folks, immigrants, and rural residents are hit hardest. Systemic inequities mean they face late diagnoses, fragmented care, higher out-of-pocket costs, and the quiet assumption they should be grateful for whatever scraps they're offered. They're the ones showing up in ERs as a last resort—not because they don't care about their health, but because every other door was "out of network" or twenty zip codes away.

Meanwhile, I had good insurance. A stable home. A supportive partner. Enough savings to float us through the worst. We didn't go into debt to pay for my treatment—but we weren't untouched.

We reviewed our budget like a set of evacuation orders—what stays, what goes. Me with sticky notes, Scott at the computer. Vacations: gone. Streaming services: gone. Takeout: gone. Our kids started hearing "not this year" more often than I wanted. I didn't want to burden anyone. But survival is a shared cost. Everyone pays.

Still, we were lucky. I know that. And honestly, that knowledge is its own kind of grief. Because no one should have to ration joy just to stay alive.

The Resume Gap No One Names

There's no elegant way to say, "I took a leave of absence to not die."

And yet, that's what many of us are expected to package neatly into a cover letter—or leave off entirely. Cancer doesn't just sabotage your body. It derails your career, fractures your momentum, and creates a resume gap hiring managers scan with raised eyebrows and zero follow-up questions.

If you're lucky, your company holds your position. If you're even luckier, it's not quietly reassigned while you're still in a hospital gown. If you've landed in the mythical HR unicorn zone, someone checks in—not to ask when you're coming back, but if you're okay.

That's not the norm.

You're told, "Take all the time you need." The subtext: Just don't expect anything to be the same.

It isn't. You return altered—physically, cognitively, emotionally—and expected to slide right back in with ease and gratitude. But chemo brain doesn't care about your calendar invites. Scar tissue doesn't love ergonomic desk chairs. And it's hard to feel "ready to re-engage" when every unknown number on your phone makes your stomach drop.

For those without sick leave, short-term disability, or an accommodating employer, the choice is even starker: work through it, or lose everything. Legal protections like FMLA or the ADA exist on paper, but they're limited, inconsistently enforced, and often inaccessible to the people who need them most.

And when you return to job searching? There's the problem of the gap.

Do I owe anyone the story of those missing years? Do I reduce my entire trauma to a line item called "medical leave"? Am I still ambitious if my only professional goal for a while was "survive"?

For me, cancer interrupted everything. I was pursuing a new career in respiratory therapy. I had to withdraw. That decision gutted me. But when the dust settled, I recalibrated. I chose something that aligned more deeply with what I'd learned: first lifestyle medicine, then social work. It wasn't a return. It was a re-rooting.

The truth is, we don't owe anyone a glossy version of what we've endured. We lived it. That's the resume line.

And honestly? If surviving cancer doesn't count as transferable experience, I don't know what does.

What the System Got Exactly Right

Cancer asked everything of me—my body, my time, my mind, my money. But it also revealed just how many invisible skills are required to survive a system like ours. You have to be a patient. A project manager. A grant writer. A policy nerd. A legal analyst. A communications strategist. A walking appointment reminder with a high pain threshold and a reliable printer.

And if you can't do all that? Hopefully you know someone who can.

On its own terms, the system got exactly what it was built for: profit protected, risk outsourced, sick people turned into line items. It got that right. It rewards those who can contort themselves into its rules and lets the rest fall through the cracks.

But healthcare shouldn't be judged by how well it shields revenue. It should be judged by how well it shields people.

Luck is not a healthcare strategy. Neither is martyrdom. The system counts on us to manage our illness without becoming a burden, to say thank you for partial access, to treat survival as a personal accomplishment instead of a collective responsibility.

I survived cancer. I also survived the system. That shouldn't be two separate accomplishments.

We deserve better than survival math.

What would healthcare look like if it began with dignity, not denial? If the default wasn't burnout and bankruptcy, but continuity and care?

I don't have all the policy answers yet. But I know this much: a system that only works if you're organized, articulate, well-insured, and endlessly persistent is not a healthcare system.

It's an obstacle course.

And sick people are not supposed to be the ones jumping the hurdles.

Emotional Buffer and Communications Strategist

Once, when I first told someone I had breast cancer, they responded with a twenty-minute story about their malfunctioning air fryer.

I had just finished explaining my diagnosis. No follow-up questions. No "How are you?" Just an immediate detour into salvaging wing night with an appliance that had, in their words, "turned on them."

When the Zoom timer cut us off, I felt nothing but relief. Scott and I just stared at each other. "That was... weird, right?" I asked.

He nodded.

That was my introduction to the idea that telling people you have cancer isn't one conversation. It's a whole communications campaign—drafts, rewrites, and aftershocks. There's a moment, right after you say the word cancer, where their face falls and suddenly you're the one comforting them.

There's no script. No optimal tone or timing. You just brace yourself, deliver the news, and hope the person on the other end doesn't crumble—or disappear.

Some reactions brought comfort: eyes that welled with love, hands that reached out without hesitation, humor timed just right to crack the tension without erasing the truth. Even when people were scared, they stayed present. They didn't make it about them.

Others... did.

Some people said nothing. Disappeared. Avoided eye contact. Changed the subject. Ghosted. I grieved those people too.

Some responses were just disorienting: blank stares, long silences, abrupt pivots to weather or shipping delays. A few people seemed to hear "I have cancer" and immediately launch into a monologue about office chairs. I kept thinking, maybe if I explain more, they'll meet me here. Sometimes they did. Sometimes they never did.

There was the friend who sobbed so hard I ended up rubbing her back. The classmate who said, "This is so hard for me to hear." The distant cousin who replied, "I just lost someone to breast cancer last year." (By the way, never volunteer this. Ever.)

I started keeping a mental list of people I needed to manage.

It didn't take long to realize I was functioning like a sponge—soaking in other people's shock, sadness, guilt, and fear. Quietly absorbing, without spilling. It felt like my job to keep them dry. Comforting. Reassuring. Holding their overwhelm while mine simmered just beneath the surface.

Even my kids, incredible and too young to be navigating this even in college, needed buffering. I chose my words carefully, stayed measured, avoided saying anything that might scare or scar them. It's a strange skill: telling the truth without telling too much.

Managing everyone else's emotions while holding my own grief was a full-time job. I became a translator, a strategist, an emotional pack mule.

Job Description: Emotional Buffer

This is the exhausting contradiction of survivorship: you're expected to be the brave one, the therapist, the tour guide through your own trauma—while still undergoing it.

Half the time, it didn't feel like I was holding back my fear; it felt like I was assigned to. To shield others from the depth of the pain I was in. To be strong. To deliver the reassuring smile and the well-practiced, "We caught it early," even on days I felt like I was dissolving by the hour.

By the time I got through that first wave of disclosures, I was already saturated. I had taken in so much—everyone else's panic, everyone else's pain. There was no space left for my own. I was heavy with it, leaking at the edges.

This was self-inflicted but not unlearned. This is what strong, modern women are trained to do, right? We don't cry at work. We don't scare the kids. We don't make our parents worry. We write the script, pick our moments, and dress up the hard parts in digestible metaphors. I translated medical jargon into Google Maps analogies, shared the good news first—always first—and saved my tears for the shower.

Only Scott was allowed into the room where I kept my fear.

If you had to put it on a résumé, it would look like this:

Role: Emotional Buffer and Communication Strategist
Employer: Everyone But Me, LLC
Dates: Diagnosis → Burnout (ongoing contract work)

Key Responsibilities:

1. Translate medical trauma into digestible, non-threatening soundbites
2. Pre-draft conversations to anticipate emotional responses and minimize collateral damage
3. Maintain upbeat tone while delivering devastating news
4. Absorb tears, gasps, awkward silences, and unsolicited prayers without retaliation
5. Uphold Strong, Independent Woman™ brand image
6. Manage internal collapse privately (see also: shower floor)

Key Skills:

1. Emotional triage
2. High-functioning dissociation
3. Smile-under-duress
4. Precision in selective disclosure
5. Boundary-setting (Advanced level, achieved mid-treatment)

Compensation: Exposure. Growth mindset. Occasional casseroles.

But here's the truth I didn't admit to myself at first: managing other people's emotions wasn't just about protecting them—it was about preserving me.

I rationed the truth based on what I could handle. Who could absorb the information without unraveling? Who would spin out and leave me to clean it up? Who would vanish, pocketing my vulnerability like a stone?

Telling the story once was hard. Telling it over and over was like re-breaking a bone to prove it still hurt.

The Interrogation Room

As if managing everyone's feelings wasn't enough, there was one question that reliably turned me from patient into confessional:

"But what caused it?"

Sometimes it came fast, as if from a script. Other times it was soft, like they knew they shouldn't ask but couldn't stop themselves. Sometimes it was curious. Other times, interrogative.

And the worst part? There was no answer. At least not one that made anyone feel better.

Genetic? Not according to my test. Environmental? Maybe. Stress? Diet? Hormones? Cell phone towers?

I don't know is the worst possible answer for people who crave certainty.

That's when I realized: they weren't really asking about me. They were asking about them.

Can I prevent this from happening to me? What makes you different from me? If I eat better, exercise more, manifest harder, can I dodge this?

It's the illusion of control. And I get it. I've chased that illusion, too.

Sometimes it felt like disbelief: "You? You're one of the healthiest people I know." Translation: If you can get cancer, maybe anyone can. Maybe I can.

Sometimes it sounded like a hunt: "Are you sure it's not from birth control? Or stress? Or the vaccine?" Like if they asked the right question, I'd finally give up the real answer.

And sometimes, it went straight to spiritual: "Everything happens for a reason." As if God runs a selective character-development program and I made the short list.

Mostly, though, people just hated the not-knowing. They hated it more than the diagnosis. Uncertainty was the real villain.

And me? I became a mirror. I reflected their fear, their need to fix, their hunger for answers. Every time I said, "I don't know," I watched disappointment wash over their faces. I couldn't give them the comfort of logic. I couldn't protect them from the randomness of it all.

So I went back to what I knew: I absorbed it. All of it.

Learning Boundaries: Wringing Out the Sponge

Cancer didn't just threaten my body. It ambushed my ability to self-regulate. I absorbed it all. Worry, silence, unsolicited advice, even grief that wasn't mine.

But slowly, I learned to wring myself out.

One of the few people who truly saw the emotional toll was my oncologist. She looked Scott in the eyes and deputized him: "Your job is to be the communicator. She needs to rest and heal."

And he did.

He wrote the email updates with compassion, clarity, and wit. Sometimes it was big—scan results, surgery dates, treatment plans. Sometimes it was just, "No news." The silence was its own form of care. It meant I didn't have to narrate my trauma on a production schedule.

There were days I couldn't open my inbox. Knowing someone else held the megaphone gave me permission to set it down. I could just be in it, without performing it.

I stopped answering every text. I left things on "read." I cancelled visits when I didn't have the emotional bandwidth to host my own pain in front of someone else's face. I chose what to share and when to share it.

I shut the faucet off on advice.

At first, I welcomed every suggestion: what to eat, which supplements, how someone's aunt's neighbor's Reiki healer cured stage 4 with essential oils and vibes. I didn't know what I didn't know, and I thought the information might empower me.

Instead, it flooded me. It contradicted itself. It made my already overloaded brain operate at a frequency only anxiety dogs could hear. I didn't need more data; I needed solid ground. Peace. Boundaries.

I also started noticing the emotional intrusions that had felt "small," but left deep internal bruises:

- Comforting people who were devastated for me while I was days from surgery.
- Answering every "How are you doing?" when what they really meant was, Please reassure me so I don't have to sit with my fear.
- Letting minimizers slide: "At least they caught it early," "You've got this," "You've had greater challenges in life." (Had I?)

Eventually, the sponge hit its limit.

The first time I typed "I don't have the capacity for this right now" and hit send, my hands shook. Nothing exploded. I let silence hang like laundry. The response: "Got it. Love you." The world kept spinning. So did I.

Boundaries, I realized, are not walls. They're doors with locks. I get to decide who comes in—and when. They give me space to breathe, to grieve, to heal. To be fully human, not just the brave patient in someone else's inspirational arc.

I wasn't strong every moment. I was just careful about when I broke.

Asking for help didn't make me weak; it made me honest.

I still catch myself reaching out, ready to absorb. But now I pause. Being soft doesn't mean being soaked. I get to decide what I carry.

And I'm done calling that strength. It's just truth.

Once I stopped managing the people who drained me, I could finally see the ones who were holding me up.

True Witnesses

There were people who needed me to be okay—quickly, cleanly, graciously. And then there were the ones who reminded me I didn't have to perform wellness to be loved.

They didn't shudder at the rawness. They didn't need a silver lining. They just showed up.

My dad and his wife became constants, no speeches required. They drove me to appointments, kept my plants alive, took my dog on a four-week adventure where he could be wild and free. They didn't ask for updates on a schedule. They didn't poke or prod. They just made space, sent their love through patient check-ins and gentle presence. No pressure to be chipper. I never once felt like a burden.

My mom, who lived out of state, came to stay with me for three weeks while Scott was away on business. She stepped into the rhythm of my days without disrupting it—helping with meals, rest, errands. One weekend, she even helped me travel to Utah to visit my step-kids. It was a gift of presence at a time when getting from point A to B felt monumental. Her being there made it possible.

Taft and Teri mailed me a care package so perfectly "me," it felt like a warm hand on my shoulder. No surprise visit. No "Let me know if you need anything." Just joy in a box—little treasures and distractions that said, *We see you*, without demanding anything in return.

Jodi, Tiff, and Jenn packed up my old house and unpacked my new one. I was in the thick of chemo, barely upright some days. They organized my fridge, scrubbed cupboards, and made sure my life could keep moving even when I couldn't. They wouldn't let me lift a finger. Somehow they made it look like the highlight of their day.

Nicole came and painted the baseboards when it was time to list the house. No fanfare. Just brushstrokes, calm conversation, and the transformation of a space I was too tired to tend.

None of these people needed anything back. That was the miracle. I didn't have to be sprightly or grateful in real time. I didn't have to curate a healing journey. I could just exist. Fragile. Foggy. Human.

They understood that love isn't always loud. Sometimes it's a ride to chemo. Sometimes it's organizing your spice rack while you nap. Sometimes it's showing up without needing to be shown anything at all.

These were my true witnesses. The ones who saw me bruised, hurting, unfinished—and stayed. Their love didn't need a performance. Their belief in me wasn't contingent on how strong I looked.

In their company, I stopped pretending I was okay. I let the sponge be heavy with everything I'd held, and they held me.

If I had to rewrite the job description I once believed came with a cancer diagnosis, it wouldn't demand endless strength, cheerful updates, or the ability to absorb everyone else's fear. It would say:

> Must be human.
>
> Must be willing to fall apart.
>
> Must learn to stop carrying what was never yours to hold.

For so long, I performed wellness like it was my duty—protecting others from my pain, sanding my truth into something smoother. Slowly, that performance cracked. I stopped being the only witness to my suffering. I let others hold parts of it with me.

In that unscripted space I discovered a kind of love that didn't ask for a mask. Just my presence. My truth. My very human self.

These days, I still wring myself out often. Gently. With care.

Being a sponge isn't strength. Let others chase heroics. I'll take whole.

Motherhood, With an IV Pole

Wholeness didn't mean life got quieter. It meant I stopped pretending I could live it in compartments.

Cancer was still there—beeping, scheduling, demanding. But so were the kids.

Motherhood didn't wait for my labs to normalize.

No Medical Leave

Jake texted me from Iowa. He was in an ophthalmologist's waiting room because a nasty infection had damaged his retina—the cat's unintended revenge for the torture she endured by being petted without permission.

"I'm literally the youngest person in this waiting room… by at least 30 years," he wrote.

I laughed. An actual, out-loud chuckle. Because I was also sitting in a doctor's office. More specifically: an infusion room. I looked up from my phone and took note of the chairs around me—hats, blankets, socks that said things like Hope and Warrior, every attempt made to bully cancer into submission through hosiery. The patients were older. The room pulsed and beeped with the occasional cough that sounded like it had been there since Nixon.

"Me too," I texted back. "By at least 30 years."

Then I told him where I was. He sent the laughing smiley-face emoji—the modern version of reaching across 800 miles and squeezing you back. For a moment, we were just two people in two medical offices, both irritated at our bodies, both trying to make it normal with humor.

The thing about motherhood during cancer was that it didn't disappear. It didn't even dim politely. No medical leave. No pause button. It just... continued. Like the background music of your life.

Available While Supplies Last

For nearly a year, my whole world was cancer. Then came the sequel—new port, surgery in a week, and a different chemo plan waiting in the wings, like the universe had me on a subscription model I did not consent to. The first version had an end date. Recurrence rewrote the schedule.

The mental fortitude was enormous. I knew I was strong enough to do it—me. But the moment I factored in my family, that's when the math got rude. In our house, "the kids" means all of them—Scott's five, my two, and the bonus kid who came with Jake. Love doesn't do footnotes.

There were only so many hours, only so much energy, and my body was making budget cuts without consulting me. My mom-default setting had always been a mix of grit and slack—high expectations with enough freedom to become themselves. Jake wanted pink hair before kindergarten; we dyed it fuchsia together because it was only hair and also, frankly, iconic. I taught them to do what they could do: laundry, chores, responsibility. We celebrated everything from birthdays to passing a spelling test. We practiced tough conversations early. I role-played conflict scripts so they could be brave without being reckless.

Then cancer showed up and said: Cute. Try this level.

By then, the kids ranged from teens to young adults—old enough to function, young enough to still want me. I couldn't relate to the mothers doing chemo with a sticky-handed three-year-old on their hip. I couldn't imagine bargaining over bedtime while bargaining with nausea.

They needed connection, advice, reassurance—because everything felt urgent and there's no know-how. They were navigating independence at full speed: new places, new responsibilities, new relationships, decisions that felt permanent because they were happening for the first time. Everything louder and closer. How to live inside their own identities. How to be safe, brave, disappointed, and keep moving. They needed hugs the way grown kids do: like they're casual about it until they're not.

I had a body that filed frequent requests for horizontal time and a life that refused to stop happening.

Some days I could do the big things: show up, parent, drive, laugh, be present. Other days I mothered the way you pack for Colorado: layers, backup plans, and a realistic relationship with the weather.

Scott and I learned the difference between the plan and what my body would allow.

He built the calendars and tracked the details—the appointments, school stuff, who needed to be where and when. Every week we'd review it together, and I'd choose the duties I thought I could carry. Then each morning he'd check in: How's your body today? Still up for this?

Most days I was. Some days I wasn't. And on the days my body pulled the plug, he covered without making it a referendum on my effort.

He made a chore chart and assigned the jobs. He meal-planned and cooked most nights, because somebody had to feed the household while I was being fed treatment after treatment.

A few weeks into that last chemo stretch, I woke up early to drive one kiddo to Denver for a girls' camping trip. I was so fatigued that morning. I created a little space through warm tea and comfy clothes. Got in the passenger seat, letting her get drive time in—hours toward her license. Together we made it to the 7 a.m. meetup point. She was excited—and her excitement was contagious.

Then I drove back up to Boulder for treatment with fifteen minutes to spare. Two and a half hours in the car, before noon, like it was my side hustle.

Another night, we went out for dinner with a couple of the kids. I wanted to see their faces. Not as proof that I was fine. As proof that I still existed outside fluorescent lighting and lab results. Cancer tried to shrink my life down to appointments and side effects. Motherhood kept insisting my life was bigger than that.

Some days I felt that collision right in my sternum—my body was trying to live one life while my children kept asking for another.

And sometimes the overlap wasn't private.

Sometimes motherhood asked me to show up in public—port, bald head, and all—like it was no big deal. Like it was just another Tuesday.

Now Appearing: Me, Unfiltered

There was a time I did cancer in public, and it felt like a costume I hadn't finished putting on—not because of what I wore, but because of what people expected to see.

It was Max's trade school graduation. Late June. The kind of morning where the sun doesn't just shine; it interrogates. We were seated on bleachers at a football field: Scott, my mom, Jake, and I. Heat radiated up from the track like the earth was exhaling. No shade. No breeze. Just the relentless, smug glare of a sky that didn't care about my white blood cell count.

I was bald from chemo, wearing it like a dare—no scarf, no hat. Just sunglasses, big hoop earrings, and a thin hooded sweater to protect my tissue paper skin. Sunscreen helped, but not enough. I looked like a very tired, very committed extra in a desert movie.

Underneath the hood, my brain was doing that rude math again. How many minutes of this heat equals one afternoon of recovery? If I pass out now, do I ruin the photos? I wasn't there to be a patient. I was there because Max had built something—a framework of discipline and pride. Watching him cross that stage, I wasn't thinking about my recurrence. I was thinking: Look at you. Look what you've made of yourself while the world was falling apart at home.

That day was about Max.

Forty-five minutes in, Max crossed the stage. He held that diploma like proof of life. I saw it, I cheered, and then my body—which had been politely waiting in the lobby—finally burst through the door and demanded a vote. My heart was thumping a frantic rhythm against my ribs. I needed shade the way a person needs air.

I stood up to slip out as quietly as I could.

The man behind me didn't know anything about my bloodwork or my scans. He just knew I was standing up. He snapped, "I watched your kid graduate. You can watch mine."

I turned to look him in the eye. I was already pulling an apology together—the reflex of a woman who who has spent a lifetime being "polite" even while her body is being dismantled. But before I could speak, his gaze dropped.

He saw the port under my collarbone. Then he saw the lack of hair beneath the hood.

He saw the math I'd been doing for the last hour. He saw that I wasn't being selfish; I was being human with a body that had reached its expiration date for the day. Shame washed over his face. He'd decided I was being disrespectful, never considering that I was surviving.

"I'm sorry," I said anyway—because old habits are harder to kill than cancer—and I moved toward the shade.

I waited, heart thumping with pride and heat. I had stayed long enough to witness him. I had spent every cent of energy I had to be there for that one walk across the stage. In the economy of cancer, that was a luxury purchase.

Motherhood didn't pause. It just kept finding me.

But if the man on the bleachers had misjudged my need to move, I was starting to misjudge my children's need to stay still.

At the hospital, time was a clinical commodity. At home, it was a moral one. I was hoarding my minutes like a survivalist, which made the math of our household feel increasingly lopsided. I started judging time by what it produced. If I was using my limited fuel to keep the world turning—to water the plants, to stay upright—I needed everyone else to be burning at the same rate.

The Obscenity of Killing Time

The problem was: I could handle hard things. What I couldn't handle was not being in charge of time. Cancer did something weird to my parenting: it made me reach for control like it was a coping skill. Not the bossy kind. The grief kind. If I couldn't control the one thing that mattered, my brain tried to manage everything else within reach.

And loving them that hard did what it always does: it made me a little unreasonable.

The place it showed up most was time.

I'd be in the kitchen, clutching the watering pitcher like a prize. I wanted to be the one watering the plants. There is something about keeping things alive when your own cells are mutinying that feels like victory.

But there was a catch: if I was working, I wanted others to be working too.

From the living room or behind closed bedroom doors, I could hear it—the rapid-fire clicking of controllers, the game music, the muffled shouts. While I was dragging my fatigue across the floor to finish one productive task, they were killing time.

To a person with a healthy prognosis, killing time is indulgence. To me, it felt like an obscenity.

I'd be standing there with the water in hand, watching the light hit the dust motes, and I'd feel a spike of hot, unreasonable resentment. I craved the things they were ignoring. I wanted the energy to go for a long walk with a friend or the stamina for a three-course meal out in the world. I was fighting for more minutes, and they were treating theirs like an infinite resource.

The friction wasn't really about the chores. It wasn't about work ethic. It was a plea: Don't waste the one thing I can't buy more of. I was treating every hour like it had an expiration date, and they were in the other room, oblivious, letting the world go gray around the edges of a monitor.

I wanted them present. I wanted them building real lives—movement, friendships, sunlight. Not because the house was a mess, but because I was terrified they were practicing disappearance just as I was being forced to leave the party early.

Every spike of anger was fear: I want you to live like I'm going to be here to see it.

Underneath it—always—was love. The kind that didn't just want to keep them safe. The kind that wanted to stay.

Which is how I ended up training for a hike like it was an argument with the universe. Not inspirational. Just stubborn.

Field Work

Eventually, the resentment over the video games would break, usually because the world outside the screen demanded a body. Mine, or theirs.

I called these moments Field Work. If treatment was the lab—sterile, controlled, and lonely—Field Work was the reality of staying woven into their lives. It was where the math of my energy met the physics of their needs.

Sometimes it looked like permanent ink.

One of the boys invited me to get matching tattoos: Mayan-inspired green sea turtles. A throwback to the trip to Akumal, a shared memory turned into a permanent connection—with the sea, the trip, and each other. We sat in the shop, the buzz of the needles a different frequency than the hum of the infusion pump. It was closeness through shared pain, but the kind that ends with art instead of a lab report. It was a way of saying: you're still my person, and I'm still here to be marked by you. And apparently: let's commemorate it with needles.

Sometimes Field Work looked like a Jeep hard top needing to be swapped before the first snow. I didn't have "lift-and-carry" energy. "I need to lie down for three business days" energy. But the Jeep was a project, and projects are the opposite of video games—they require gravity and tools and grease. I couldn't lift the roof, but I could be a stabilizer. I leaned my weight into the frame, steadying the heavy plastic while he fumbled with the hardware.

I was a human sandbag, maternal edition.

There's a specific kind of brave nobody claps for: the kind that just holds the line so the bolt can finally catch the thread. In that moment, leaning against the cold metal, I wasn't a woman with a recurrence. I was just a mom helping her son winterize his life.

Then there was the long haul: Iowa to Colorado to Albuquerque.

A car loaded with the debris of a new beginning—leafy plants and a kitchen box labeled UTENSILS. My job was the "Consultant of the Ordinary." I drove, I picked out plants for a garden, and I navigated the first-weekend-of-a-new-life chaos.

I taught him how to use a gas grill and how to sear salmon so it didn't turn into pencil erasers. It sounds small until you realize it's the whole point: a kid building a life, and me refusing to be edited out of it. I was teaching, laughing, and insisting on protein.

This is what survival looks like from the inside. It's the stubborn refusal to let the subscription model of cancer cancel your membership in the mundane.

Carrots, Electrolytes, and Character Development

The culmination of all this math and field work happened on a trail.

I was training for a big hike with Scott and the girls—seven miles, two thousand feet of elevation gain. I was determined. I was also slow. While they had their easy banter going, my focus was embarrassingly basic: breathe, step, breathe, step. Keep one foot in front of the other. Try not to turn this family hike into an unscheduled cardiology consult.

When the trail got steep, I had to stop. I'd stand there with my hands on my poles, waiting for my heart rate to come back down into a range that didn't feel like a personal insult. I drank electrolytes like they were a life force. I ate a small bag of carrots to keep my blood sugar from doing anything creative. Then I started again. Trudge. Breathe. Repeat.

After an hour of this uphill negotiation, one of the girls looked back at me and said, almost casually, "You're an inspiration."

It just about knocked the wind out of my lungs. Not because it was profound, but because she wasn't asking me to perform anything. She wasn't looking at a Warrior sock or a pink ribbon. She was just noticing the math of the climb.

That's the only kind of "inspiration" I'll accept: witnessed by someone who loves me, with no audience.

Cancer wanted my whole identity. It tried to make my world small. The kids kept interrupting with things like real life—Jeep tops, tattoos, graduation caps, and Iowa waiting rooms. I appreciate them for the inconvenience.

Motherhood didn't pause—it just kept finding me. It came in texts. It came in beeps. It came in the spaces between.

PART III

The Afterbody

When Your Liver Taps Out & Your Toes Need Surgery

It started with my toes—red, fleshy blisters, impossibly tender. Something as small as nail pain shouldn't feel like collapse, but it did. Turns out, they'd had enough.

Over two years into active treatment, I was on Xeloda, an oral chemotherapy drug prescribed after I completed radiation. It was part of a layered treatment plan designed to keep my aggressive breast cancer from coming back. Because of my recurrence and the presence of mixed cancer cells, my oncologist wanted to throw everything we had at it. Xeloda is known for targeting cancer cells more selectively than traditional chemo, but it still comes with its own charming list of side effects.

At the top of that list? Hand and Foot Syndrome. A condition that sounds almost cute—until your skin starts blistering, peeling, and turning the color of a ripe tomato. It's caused by chemo leaking into the capillaries of your palms and soles, irritating the tissues and eventually making basic tasks like walking or opening a jar feel like medieval punishment. To get ahead of it, I was told to apply Udder Cream, a balm originally designed for cow udders, because that's where we're at now, slathered generously on my hands and feet. On top of that, I was instructed to layer in Voltaren, an anti-inflammatory gel to treat pain and inflammation.

Pro tip: don't use a topical medication you're allergic to while soaking your skin in cow lotion and taking oral chemo.

Turns out, I had a sensitivity to one of the active ingredients in Voltaren. My immune system was already working overtime, and the gel pushed it over the edge. The skin around my toes became inflamed, cracked, and eventually opened. The pain was sharp and constant. My podiatrist looked at them and said, "It's not Hand and Foot Syndrome exactly... more like a highly localized uprising."

He wasn't wrong. My toes had simply reached the end of their ability to cooperate.

They were bleeding daily, a slow seep until a light bump would trigger a ten-minute hemorrhage. Surgery on both big toes was required. My toenails had basically mutated. Chemo had not only altered their color, but also their growth pattern, causing them to curl into the skin like little saboteurs. "Like an ingrown toenail, but worse," he said cheerfully. "We'll need to remove part of the tissue and reshape the nail bed."

I nodded like I was ordering Chipotle. Just one more surreal item on the cancer errand list: radiation burns, immunotherapy infusion, ovary ousting, toe debridement. No big deal.

Except it was.

As I sat there, nodding and pretending this was normal, something cracked open. Not in my toes—those were already split wide. In my understanding of what my body had been trying to tell me. For months I'd ignored the whispers. This time, it screamed through my digits: We're tired. We can't keep doing this.

After my surgery, the podiatrist handed me aftercare instructions and a prescription for antibiotics like it was no big deal, but I left the office blinking back a surprising wave of grief. And relief. The pain was finally being addressed. This was a step (ha.) toward healing. Forward motion. My body had been waving the white flag for weeks, and someone had finally noticed. But that progress didn't cancel out the ache. Instead, the two feelings lived side by side: the gratitude of being helped and sorrow that I'd needed help in the first place.

This was something else. Subtler. Deeper. It was about weariness. About having to pretend that each new breaking point was just another box to tick on the cancer care checklist. My body wasn't breaking down from cancer. It was breaking down from the cure. You expect cancer to be the villain, not the treatment.

But this? This wasn't cancer coming for me. This was the aftermath of every drug, every infusion, every aggressive, well-intentioned assault on my cells. My toes were simply the first ones to tap out.

I didn't arrive at that silence on my own. I'd been coached into it.

The Warrior Myth and Its Collateral Damage

The first time someone called me a warrior, I didn't have a clue how to respond. It was early in the journey, back when I still believed there would be a clean line between treatment and recovery, before I learned that survival would look more like a game of medical whack-a-mole than a victorious finish line.

People meant well, of course. *You're so strong. So brave. A total badass. You've got this.* The subtext was always the same: keep going. Don't falter. Keep performing your strength; it reassures us. It lets us believe you're okay, because we don't always know what to do with someone else's pain.

And I did. For a long time.

I cracked jokes about drains and chemo. I sent upbeat email updates. I filtered my pain into palatable soundbites. I brushed past constipation that lasted weeks, gut cramps that left me face down on the floor, muscle wasting, skin peeling, and a body I barely recognized anymore. Those things didn't fit the narrative of triumph. They didn't belong in the gift-shop version of survivorship.

In one of my support groups, a woman pointed out that we're socialized to smile through pain, to hide the raw parts. She likened it to postpartum recovery: all celebration, no stitches. All baby joy, no sobbing on the bathroom floor at 3 a.m.

That conversation was the first time I really asked myself: What's the cost of always being strong?

For me, it was numbness. Detachment. The subtle, creeping erosion of self-trust. Because if strength is the only acceptable language, what do you do with fear? With ambivalence? With fatigue so thick you start building exit routes into your vacation plans "just in case"?

When I finally started to name those feelings—grief, uncertainty, frustration, shame—it wasn't weakness. It was authentic. I wasn't failing. I was finally telling the truth.

The Accumulation: How Much Is Too Much?

The thing about cancer treatment is that it seemingly never ends. It evolves. Morphs. Adds layers. It's not a one-time exorcism; it's a prolonged occupation. And over time, even the most resilient body begins to protest.

By the time my liver joined the rebellion, I had been on some form of active treatment for nearly three years. Immunotherapy, oral and infusion chemos, monthly ovarian suppression shots, hormone blockers, physical therapy, acupuncture, radiation, targeted therapy, too many surgeries to count, and every blood draw, scan, supplement, and sunscreen reminder in between. I tracked it all. An entire spreadsheet to manage the onslaught—loud in its chaos, invisible on the surface. I was meticulous. Organized. Committed.

And yet, I couldn't outrun the accumulation. My skin burned from radiation. My muscles atrophied from months of inactivity. My brain fog was so thick I forgot the word for doorknob. The structure of my nails had literally changed, warped by repeated chemo exposure, curling into the surrounding tissue like tiny, inflamed blades.

And then came the labs.

My bloodwork lit up with a new red flag: liver toxicity. The targeted therapy I'd been taking, ribociclib, was designed to block proteins that help cancer cells multiply. A good idea in theory. In practice, it was now actively harming my liver.

We paused the medication. Let my body recover. Steroids helped. It took two months for my liver to heal. I resumed on a lower dose. Within a week, the damage returned. My oncologist stated this wasn't sustainable. My body made that decision.

When I looked at her and said, "My liver's saying enough. What's next?" she didn't argue. She agreed. I was recognized for having followed every direction and for having a body that had simply taken one more hit than it could handle. It felt... complicated.

The nausea, fatigue, and vomiting I'd been chalking up to stress or general cancer exhaustion suddenly made sense. It wasn't that I was weak, it was that my internal organs were literally shutting down pieces of themselves in order to survive the cure. The irony was as sharp as the pain: the thing keeping me alive might also be the thing that breaks me.

There was no dramatic moment of collapse. No ambulance or emergency room. Just a slow, steady realization that I could not keep saying yes to everything. Not without consequence.

This wasn't giving up. This was getting honest.

Disruption Fatigue: Body, Mind, Identity

Surviving cancer often means living inside a rolling state of disruption. It's not just physical. It's logistical, emotional, relational, even spiritual. The disruptions show up in the mailbox, on the calendar, in the mirror, and in your sense of self.

I used to believe that treatment was a detour. A pause for temporary construction. Something I'd push through and emerge from, sweaty and triumphant. But cancer doesn't work like that. Treatment isn't a mile marker. It's a whole new city. And after months of reroutes and recalculations—side effects, setbacks, system navigation—I started to forget what life felt like before I spoke in acronyms: PET, MRI, CBC, ER+, TNBC.

There was a moment I caught my reflection and didn't recognize it. Short, wiry hair. Loose skin in my arms. New scars that didn't follow a surgical line but bloomed unpredictably. Fatigue that no amount of sleep could touch. My face looked ten years older. My body didn't feel like mine. It felt like a rental, unfamiliar, dinged up, with a warning light I was told to ignore.

And it wasn't just the body. It was the life I had imagined living.

I'd spent months recalibrating everything: school on pause, career transitions derailed, vacations rewritten with escape routes. I stopped buying tickets more than two weeks in advance. Everything became a maybe. A tentative RSVP to my own future.

There's a term in the medical journals—cancer-related fatigue. To borrow the definition from the American Cancer Society, cancer-related fatigue is "a physical, emotional, and mental feeling of tiredness or exhaustion in someone with cancer. This feeling doesn't get better with rest or sleep." But what I felt was something deeper.

If cancer-related fatigue is what happens to your cells, disruption fatigue is what happens to your life.

For me, it was the chronic state of planning with an asterisk. Of rewriting my calendar around scans and side effects. Of living under the shadow of an unreliable narrator—my own body. I was trying to rebuild a life while still actively being disassembled. It's a strange kind of existence.

I kept wondering: How do you live a meaningful life when it has to be structured around constant medical caveats? How do you keep reaching forward when your body keeps sabotaging the terms?

No, Actually, I'm Done Now... Maybe?

The second time my liver screamed at me, I heard it. Loud and clear.

It wasn't just the elevated enzymes. It was fatigue that blanketed everything. The dull nausea that made food unappealing. The way my brain stopped generating ideas. My body felt like it had been drained of all ambition, curiosity, and spark. It was as if my cells were whispering: Please. Stop.

So I did. I stopped the ribociclib. The drug is not for me.

Saying no felt radical. Not because I'm defiant, but because I had been so damn obedient. I followed every direction. I showed up to every appointment. Took every pill. Tolerated every side effect. I did it all.

Until I didn't.

This wasn't a failure of discipline or a lack of willpower. This was self-preservation. This was reclamation. This was the moment I realized that healing isn't always about compliance. Sometimes, it's about consent. About knowing when to pivot. And about listening better—to science and to myself. I wasn't stepping back. I was stepping into a different kind of power. The power of discernment; reclaiming my body from a system that too often saw it as a site of risk rather than a place of life.

Saying no isn't the end of the conversation. No doesn't mean never. It just means not this, not now, not at that cost. I turned down ribociclib, but I haven't turned my back on treatment. There's another drug, with different risks and trade-offs, and I'm considering it. Not out of fear. But because I now know how to weigh the cost. Because I finally trust myself to choose.

There's no spreadsheet that can tell you exactly how much protection you're trading for how much pain. Only probabilities, educated guesses, and your own threshold for what a life is worth living in.

What followed wasn't a sensational montage of immediate relief. It was a slow, strange stillness—the kind of in-between that allows for a slightly deeper breath.

Healing Without Heroics

For a while, I thought healing would feel like success. The kind of thing you announce, pose with, hashtag.

Instead, it felt like... elbow room.

It crept in slowly, like light through a cracked window—gentle, soft, almost imperceptible. After I stopped ribociclib and my body had a chance to exhale, something in me loosened. Not everything. The fatigue was still there. So was the brain fog, the lymphedema. But there was space. Not just in my calendar or my bloodstream, but in my mind.

It caught me off guard during a healing touch session. I'd gone in with mild skepticism, expecting little more than an hour of rest. But something in the music, the tranquility, the warmth—something in that moment let me feel awe. Not inspiration, not adrenaline. Awe. A deep, profound appreciation for the sheer range of emotion I had survived.

I thought about all the times I had spiraled, numbed, endured. And how, in retrospect, every single emotion had taught me something true. I had become emotionally fluent in a way I never imagined possible. I could name more than just the usual suspects—sad, mad, fine. I had learned to recognize grief not as an intruder, but as a houseguest. That exhaustion doesn't need justification. That silence isn't absence—it's an answer. That saying no doesn't mean giving up. It means finally trusting yourself enough to stop begging your body to earn its worth.

No one claps for this kind of healing. There are no bells to ring. No hashtags. No staged smiles. Just soft clothes, hydrating serums, a warm hand on your own back. And enough grace to forgive your reflection when you don't recognize her.

This wasn't heroism. This was being human.

And maybe, after everything, that's enough.

Choosing Life (with Caveats)

I'm still in maintenance mode. Still doing blood draws. Still monitored closely by a medical team that trusts me when I say, "Something's off." The difference now is that all of it—every scan, pill, and pause—happens as a partnership. I've learned to walk with treatment decisions. Carefully. Discerningly. Willingly.

I would love to say I've taken an early retirement from my cancer career. The hours were punishing, the benefits mixed, and the dress code—frankly—was aggressive. I've updated my résumé to include "part-time overachiever in cell mutation management" and "freelance navigator of complex systems with unreliable equipment." I've also learned to clock out, to let my body rest without apology, to leave some messages unanswered.

My toes have mostly forgiven me. The nail beds are still weird; so am I.

What's next? I don't know exactly. More scans. A new medication—rumored to come with spectacularly ill-timed diarrhea, which is not high on my wish list, except for the tiny part of me that just wants my bowels to remember how to move again. Another surgery. Another pivot, or two, or ten.

But also: more laughter, more softness, more weekends where nothing hurts and no one pokes me with a needle. More space to live in a body that doesn't have to perform heroism to deserve care.

Because that's what this has been all along—not a fight to the death, but a practice in choosing life. With nuance. With boundaries. With myself intact.

And maybe, if I'm lucky, with ten healthy toes.

Maintenance Mode, Maximum Effort

Welcome to Maintenance Mode (No One Brings Balloons)

Three years into survivorship, it's not that I've found clarity. It's that I've stopped looking for it in the places people told me to. This phase isn't about reclaiming a past life—it's about inhabiting a new one. It's less rebirth, more weird sequel. There's no makeover montage.

Just me and my calendar alerts for bone density scans, trying not to schedule joy and lab work on the same day. No post-treatment pink parade. Just me hunched over a medication tracker, trying to remember if I took my calcium supplement.

They call it maintenance mode, like it's a gentle, low-stakes phase. Unmentioned is the "maximum effort" clause.

Survivorship feels more like an unmarked trail through overgrown terrain. The body is no longer in crisis, but it's still making demands. My schedule is lighter, but my brain hasn't caught on. I still wake up scanning for symptoms. Still recoil at certain smells—rubbing alcohol, surgical tape, whatever they use to sterilize fear. The adrenaline has faded, but the muscle memory lingers.

Energy as a Rationed Commodity

I used to think maintenance mode meant cured. It doesn't. It means life continues under medical surveillance. It means planning your week around energy like it's a rationed commodity. It means every invitation requires a small risk assessment. It means explaining to your calendar why you can't have a dentist appointment and a social life in the same 48 hours.

People expect a return to normal after cancer. What I've returned to is a life restructured by boundaries—hard-won, essential, and sometimes misunderstood. I say no more often now. Dodge emotional vampires. Leave group texts on mute indefinitely.

It's not antisocial. It's self-preservation. Hermiting has become an act of reclamation. A way of honoring the body that has carried me through, the mind still healing, and the spirit that refuses to spend its limited energy explaining things to people who don't—or won't—get it.

Sometimes healing looks like a day with nothing expected of you. Sometimes it looks like showing up carefully, on purpose.

Several days after my toe surgery, I went to a Colorado Rapids game with my husband and stepdaughter. It was the Fourth of July, and the stadium was packed, a fireworks show scheduled after the game. I walked a little more delicately than usual, trying to keep an invisible buffer around my feet. The idea of someone stepping on my freshly debrided toes was enough to make me break out in a nervous sweat.

I almost never drink soda, but I celebrated with a Coke Zero. Both Kelly and Scott did a double take, like I'd just announced I was taking up professional ice dancing. The concourse was loud and crowded—music blaring, a mini-fair with rides, games, and fried everything. We skipped all of it and found a patch of shade under a tree, spreading a blanket on the grass.

The weather was perfect. Sunny. My hair had finally reached the middle of my ears—awkward, weird, very curly. Not a style anyone chooses on purpose. My eyebrows had grown back. Cancer's visual signature was fading, but my body still felt off-balance. Lymphedema was just starting to flare in my right arm, tugging at my sense of symmetry.

I tried to put all that background noise behind me and just enjoy my shady spot and my people. Pink sunglasses on my face, lenses reflecting warm swirls of oranges and pinks. A random guy walking past stopped to compliment my shades, told me they were "seriously cool," and kept going.

It was one of the first moments I remember being seen as myself again, not as a cancer patient.

The Coke Zero was a one-and-done experiment; I switched back to water as soon as I finished it. A few short weeks later, I was back under bright lights for surgery to remove my ovaries, nested in a flurry of appointments—oncology, breast surgeon, OB, pick a specialty, any specialty. A couple of months after that came another revision surgery.

This is what passes for balance now: one eye on the medical machine, the other on whatever still feels human.

When the Noise Stops and the Echoes Start

When treatments ended—at least the big, dramatic ones—everyone around me let out a collective exhale, breathing a sigh of relief. I didn't.

I celebrated, sure. There was a burst of delight. Then it ground to a halt with the realization that surgery led to chemo. Chemo to radiation. Radiation back to chemo. Chemo to targeted therapy. Endocrine and immunotherapy threaded throughout. Each chapter blurred into the next, the promised "after" always slightly out of reach.

I lived from appointment to appointment for over three years. Then one day the rhythm slowed. And in the silence, I noticed the ache.

I still remember the burns of radiation on my chest and back. The way my skin smelled faintly scorched for weeks. But the stillness? That comes out of nowhere. The aftershocks of trauma that don't show up in bloodwork. The vigilance that keeps you scanning your body like a radar dish.

The lingering that clouds your memory. The pain that pinches at odd hours. The strange way you feel like a guest in your own skin. How breast cancer still crosses your mind every damn day—sometimes faintly, sometimes like a freight train.

The Unglamorous Job of Staying Alive

Maintenance mode is what happens when the crisis ends but the work doesn't. There's nothing passive about it. I'm still monitored. Still managing medications—nine, at last count. Still doing monthly blood draws. Still slipping on my compression sleeve, booking physical therapy, watching my electrolytes and sun exposure and bone density and mood.

The term suggests stability, but there's nothing secure about it. The side effects are more benign, but they're sneakier. Fatigue arrives disguised as disinterest. Brain fog makes me question if I'm losing my mind or just tired. My days are a part-time job in symptom management and emotional project planning. There's no medal for this kind of labor, just a drawer full of co-pay receipts and a spreadsheet of symptoms. And the hope that the next blood panel doesn't throw a curve ball.

Maintenance mode isn't recovery. It's vigilance with better lighting.

Co-Writing the Plan (Without a Script)

Medical language has changed, too. Early on, it was prescriptive. There was a plan—grueling, but clear. I signed my name under a list of treatments and did my best to survive them.

Back then, I didn't have to invent the next step. The path was brutal, but it was paved. Infusion on this day. Labs on that day. Surgery scheduled. Radiation mapped. Even the fear had a calendar.

Now I'm asked to co-author a script I can't see.

"What do you want to do?" they ask, as if there's a right answer I just haven't studied for. As if there's a syllabus for living in the long middle. As if I can check out a library book titled *How to Choose the Correct Amount of Risk for the Rest of Your Life.*

Sometimes I have an opinion. Sometimes I even have a strong one. I've earned preferences the hard way—through side effects, through fatigue, through the strange intimacy of living in a body with a medical file. But sometimes I wish someone would just tell me again. Not because I want to be controlled.

Because decision-making, when every option has asterisked consequences, is its own kind of exhaustion.

Shared decision-making sounds empowering until you're the one holding the pen.

It means translating percentages into sleep, into libido, into bone density, into mood. It means weighing recurrence risk against the version of yourself you're able to inhabit. It means hearing, "We can continue," or "We can pause," or "We can switch," and realizing that none of those verbs come with certainty—just different tradeoffs and different kinds of waiting.

Early on, even bad news was clearer than this in-between. At least then, the question was mostly *Can I endure it?* Now the question is *Which consequences am I willing to live with?* That's a subtler dilemma, and somehow heavier. There's no bell for choosing. No parade for opting in or opting out. No clear moment where you're allowed to feel brave about it.

Without the rhythm of weekly appointments, without the adrenaline of crisis, I'm often unmoored. The gaps between care are supposed to feel like freedom, but they can feel like being left alone with the variables. And when someone asks me what I want to do next, I hear the real question underneath it: *Who are you now, when you're not actively surviving?*

Two Timelines, One Body

I tried rejoining the world once. I took a pottery class. It got interrupted by a recurrence. I went on a road trip. I scheduled lymph node surgery from a picnic table at a national park. The park ranger was talking about trail conditions while I was mentally mapping operating room availability.

A couple of months later, we flew to Iowa for a long weekend to visit my son at school. We hung out with him, his partner, and their roommates. One afternoon we went to an apple orchard and picked fruit straight off the trees, eating as we went, juice running down our wrists to our elbows. The stickiness disappeared under how ridiculously good those apples were.

We went to the homecoming game, where his partner was cheerleading. They won. We sprawled in his apartment between events, eating takeout while I snuck in naps I pretended were "just resting my eyes."

On our last morning together, we walked the 5K I wrote about earlier. Another small milestone disguised as a casual family event. To anyone watching, we looked like any other group crossing the finish line. Inside, I was doing the math on meds, stamina, and the nearest bathroom.

Time got erratic. The days between scans felt both too short and endless, like I was always either recovering from news or waiting for it.

My life now exists in dual timelines: the visible one where I make plans, and the hidden one where I'm always a little bit braced. Always mapping the closest exit, always aware of which arm can't take blood pressure, which veins to save, how far I am from a chair.

Too Well to Be Sick, Too Altered to Be Well

When things finally slowed down, my thoughts didn't.

During the worst of treatment, I could barely keep up. There wasn't time to wonder who had vanished or why; I was too busy surviving the next appointment, the next side effect, the next scan. Maintenance mode changed the tempo. Suddenly, everything around me felt like it was moving in slow motion, and there was just enough quiet to notice the empty chairs.

With more space came more stories. Did they care and not know how to say it? Did they move on because I'd been sick for two years and was no fun anymore? Did I make it too hard to stay close?

It was brutal trying to hold compassion for other people's limits while my own heart ached in this tender, remorseful way. I could understand why someone might pull back from the intensity of my life and still feel gutted that they had. Both were true.

During this time, I realized how many conversations with the people who *did* show up started the same way: "How are you doing? What's the game plan now?"

I became a one-woman press conference. I'd run through the latest scan, the current meds, the next follow-up, like a record playing the same track over and over. Each time I told the story, it wore down a little more. Tiny pops and scratches started to interrupt the song.

When the update was over, there was that abrupt lift of the needle—conversation finished—only for it to drop back down the next time someone asked. Same song. Same groove. A little more static every time.

After a while, I wasn't just tired of talking about cancer. I was tired of hearing myself talk about cancer. I felt like a droning talking head, the world's least entertaining podcast. There were days I didn't want to be around me either.

It's a strange kind of solitude—too well to be sick, too altered to be well, and too exhausted by the story to keep narrating it out loud.

Progress Without Fireworks

Progress is no longer climactic. It's walking five flat miles without planning my route around benches. It's remembering a word without playing charades with myself. It's cooking dinner and having the energy to stay awake for a movie.

It's noticing that the burn is now a scar, and the scar is no longer angry.

Maintenance mode isn't a return. It's a continuation. A simpler kind of living —still real, still work, just less theatrical. No fireworks. No finale. Just one step forward, and then another, lit only by the lamp I carry myself.

This is the unglamorous heart of survivorship. Not winning. Not losing. Just living. Maintenance mode doesn't ask for applause. It asks for endurance—unseen, relentless, and never quite done.

Just me—still here. Still showing up. Still building the small, stubborn rituals that keep this life livable, and keep the rage and joy from taking the wheel.

Rage, Joy, and the Ritual of Ringing the Damn Bell

Raging Against the Bell

Rituals are supposed to make meaning. Instead, I find myself ringing a brass bell bolted to the radiation oncology wall like I'm a cruise ship passenger celebrating towel animals and shuffleboard. A nurse applauds. Someone claps a little too loudly. Cheers echo down the hallway.

A woman who just got diagnosed walks past me on her way to the waiting room. I ring the damn bell because that's what you're supposed to do. Because people need the photo.

Because otherwise, what was it all for?

They say rituals mark transitions. But what if the transition isn't clean? What if it's not a crossing, but a circling? What if you step through the ceremonial doorway only to find a hallway that never ends?

We're told that closure is possible. That celebration is a choice. That the confetti at the end of treatment is made of healing. But the truth is tricky. Sometimes joy feels like a betrayal. Relief is tainted with guilt. You can't celebrate while grieving the parts of you that didn't survive. And you can't grieve out loud while everyone's cheering.

A Partial List of Rituals I Didn't Want to Do

1. Ring the bell: I did.
2. Wear a pink tutu at a breast cancer walk: I didn't.
3. Post the triumphant selfie: I did, with some less flattering but honest selfies too.
4. Pretend this was ever linear: I tried, unintentionally.
5. Smile while someone tells me "you got this": all the goddamned time.

Rituals can be powerful when they're chosen. But when they're imposed, they become performance. And no one performs harder than a woman with cancer who doesn't want to make anyone uncomfortable.

Sometimes I screamed in the shower. Sometimes I screamed at the insurance company's website. Sometimes I didn't scream at all, because I was too busy writing thank-you notes.

They say I'm brave. I say I'm tired.

They say I'm an inspiration. I say I'm managing other people's feelings with a port in my chest.

They say I should celebrate. I say I'm still in treatment. (But I think they might be right on this one.)

They say I'm done. I say, *am I?*

I Am Not Your Hallmark Card

We talk about "mixed feelings" like they're polite. What I had was emotional whiplash: rage, gratitude, grief, relief, dread, all trying to share one cramped waiting room in my chest.

If Hallmark wrote a card for that, it might look like this:

Emotional Paradoxes, Rendered in Greeting Card Format

(With deepest apologies to Hallmark)

Front of the Card:

Thinking of You During This Difficult Time

(A delicate watercolor of a pink ribbon draped over a sunset)

Inside Left:

Some days you cry, some days you fight,
Some days your soul slips out of sight.
You're brave, you're scared, you rage, you rest,
You fake a smile, you do your best.

They want neat lines, clean arcs, and cheer,
But grief and hope both camp out here.
You're stronger than they understand,
Still soft enough to hold your hand.

Inside Right:

But let's be honest.

If I get through this with my organs and my sense of humor intact, that's not resilience.

That's goddamn wizardry.

Don't tell me I'm a warrior.
Don't hand me a cupcake and call it closure.
Don't show me a bell and call it healing.

And for the love of all the gods,
I am not your fucking Hallmark card.

Making My Own Rituals

Ritual, it turns out, is where my rage and joy could sit in the same room without canceling each other out. If the prescribed rituals don't fit, you don't have to throw out the idea of ritual entirely. You just start smaller. Closer to the bone.

This is my ritual:

- I light a candle on days I need warmth in my soul.
- I wear the same soft "Fuck Cancer" socks to every infusion.
- I exhale before every test result.
- I sit in my car after every appointment and breathe like I'm resuscitating my own humanity.
- Sometimes I talk to my body, thanking it for surviving.
- Other times I sit in silence, honoring the parts that didn't.

There are no cupcakes in that ceremony, sadly.

Healing doesn't arrive with confetti. It arrives in fragments. In maintenance mode, there are no big milestones left, just blood draws and follow-ups. Rituals became how I marked time when the calendar felt like an endless grid. Those fragments looked like: a haircut that feels like a comeback; a moment of peace in a dressing room lit like a surgical suite; a friend saying, "You don't owe me a smile."

It arrives in dry humor and crisp mornings and the body remembering how to want things again.

Healing arrives in rebellion, too. In saying no to pinkwashed performance. In refusing to package your grief in gift wrap. In writing your own damn ending, even if it's still unfolding.

So yes, I rang the bell. Like last call at a dive bar.

But I also made my own ritual: a playlist. A painting. A whispered "fuck you" to the hallway of endless scans. A toast to joy and a refusal—fierce and necessary—to be anyone's Hallmark card.

Not all important moments come with a hashtag or a bell. Some arrive in T-shirts and ticket stubs. Illness took many things, but it never took the music.

Joy as Counter-Ritual

The same day as my initial biopsy, our family went to see OneRepublic. My right boob had two core samples suctioned from it in the morning so dancing that evening was out of the question. But I stood there, wincing through the pain, and sang my heart out. Loud. Off-key. Present.

The night before my mastectomy, Scott and I sat under a painted Colorado sky, letting Jack Johnson's mellow tunes wash over us. The crowd was chill, the sunset was velvet. I clung to the moment like it was a lullaby.

Three days post-mastectomy—still stitched, drained, and padded—we went to Imagine Dragons. I was held together by a compression bra and nerve block, the weather was perfect and the stage electric. It was my second time seeing them, Scott's first. The music pulsed through me like defiance. Drains and all, I was alive in the crowd.

Five days before my lymph node dissection, I took the girls (in a book focused on boobs this can be confusing—I mean my best friends here) to see lovely.the.band. One of my favorites. One of *our* favorites. We sang, we jumped, we claimed the night as ours.

And then there was Red Rocks. First day of chemo, round two, course two. Recurrence. Our friends had invited us—one of them navigating her own breast cancer chapter. It felt like a vivid act of solidarity, a way of saying, "Let's be here. Let's feel this." Our seats were second row center for Nathaniel Rateliff & the Night Sweats. The passion, the grit, the sweat and soul pouring off that stage—it reminded me of what it means to be fully alive, even when poison literally coursed through my veins.

To bear witness and to be witnessed. To let joy have a place in the middle of uncertainty.

Concerts didn't ease my treatments or my trauma. But they anchored me in time. They said: *You are here. You are still here.* And sometimes, that was enough.

We talk so much about surviving, enduring, pushing through. But there's another kind of ritual—one that sings, not shouts. One that reminds you what it feels like to be lit up from the inside, to feel rhythm in your chest that isn't fear or arrhythmia but music.

Survival wasn't always clinical. Sometimes it was dancing in place while your drains bounced with the beat.

Because the rituals that matter most are the ones that help us stay human.

They can keep the cupcake. I'll take the concert ticket, the sarcasm, the silence, and the socks. I didn't get closure. But I did get one hell of a soundtrack.

At some point, I started keeping a list—songs that held my rage, my grief, my stubborn joy. Not as a cure. As a record. Eventually, the lists expanded—beyond playlists and into the rest of my life.

Liner Notes from the Long Haul

A soundtrack for the long middle, the tumultuous rebuild, and dancing with drains.

You don't have to know any of these songs. You just have to know there was always a soundtrack—a bassline beneath the chaos—even on the days I couldn't hear it yet.

1. **"I Wanna Get Better"** – Bleachers
   Because sometimes breaking is the beginning.
2. **"The Night We Met"** – Lord Huron
   For the parts of you that didn't make it.
3. **"Just a Girl"** – No Doubt
   For every time you had to smile while someone told you to "stay positive."
4. **"Better Together"** – Jack Johnson
   Peace before the storm.
5. **"You Don't Own Me"** – Lesley Gore
   The ultimate boundary-setting anthem.
6. **"Coachella"** – lovely.the.band
   Beautifully disillusioned.
7. **"Dog Days Are Over"** – Florence + the Machine
   A joy so fierce it feels like protest.

8. **"(Don't Fear) The Reaper"** – Blue Öyster Cult
Making friends with the shadow.
9. **"Counting Stars"** – OneRepublic
Biopsy day. I sang my damn heart out.
10. **"Silver Lining"** – Mt. Joy
Hope threaded through grit and surrender.
11. **"Electric Feel"** – MGMT
Proof that electricity isn't just for nerve pain.
12. **"Unsteady"** – X Ambassadors
For every moment you tried to stand in a body that wasn't cooperating.
13. **"Flaws"** – Bastille
Radical acceptance—owning every crack in the mirror.
14. **"First"** – Cold War Kids
For when you start writing your own story again.
15. **"Stargazing"** – Myles Smith
Tender and hopeful, a soft return to dreaming.
16. **"Heat Waves"** – Glass Animals
Grief and desire in a warm synth hug.
17. **"Cardiac Arrest"** – Bad Suns
For the first time you feel alive and a little dangerous again.
18. **"Whatever It Takes"** – Imagine Dragons
Drains bouncing to the beat. Literally.
19. **"S.O.B."** – Nathaniel Rateliff & the Night Sweats
Red Rocks. Row 2. Magic.
20. **"The Mother We Share"** – CHVRCHES
Holy noise for the unholy mess.
21. **"Glitter & Gold"** – Barns Courtney
Digging for the shine underneath the rubble.

22. **"Movement"** – Hozier
A gorgeous, sweeping finale—grounded and wide-open—like being reminded you still have a pulse and a future.

You'll Want a Spreadsheet for That

Why This Matters

By the time I'd built a soundtrack for my cancer life, I realized I needed something else too: a way to keep track of the pandemonium on paper.

I was trying to tell the same story to nine different people—each one holding a clipboard. Each one asked the same questions with slightly different wording, like they'd all been assigned the same group project and refused to share notes.

"When was your last MRI?" "What kind of chemo are you currently on?" "Have you had any allergic reactions to medication?"

I wanted to sound consistent. Informed. Capable. Not like someone who had cried that morning over a yogurt lid because it said peach and I was certain I'd bought plain.

I didn't want to fall apart in front of them. I didn't want to be the fragile one, the "poor thing," the patient whose chart got annotated with soft voices and extra pamphlets. I wanted to know things about my own body. I wanted to answer quickly, like I belonged in the room.

And I did know—sort of. I just couldn't access the information in real time, not while sitting on a cold exam table, wearing a paper shirt, and trying to remember if I'd already told this doctor about the allergic reaction or if that was the other one with the similar haircut.

That's when it clicked: having a system isn't just about being organized. It's something to grab when everything else is moving.

It's a way to remember who you are and what you've already survived when the details start to smear. And they will smear. This isn't just a treatment plan. This is your life, sliced into appointments and acronyms. And it's okay to want a little order in the lawlessness.

Analog Survival

I didn't start with a spreadsheet. I started with a small spiral-bound notebook that fit in my purse.

It felt doable. Not intimidating. Not color-coded. Just paper and a pen and the hope that if I wrote things down, I might not lose them.

At the front, I reserved a few pages for the information I kept getting asked for on repeat: doctor names, diagnosis details, pathology jargon, phone numbers, office locations. The phrases I stumbled over the most got their own line, spelled correctly, underlined.

The rest of the notebook became a log. Each appointment got its own page: date, time, which specialist, clinic address. Before I went in, I'd jot down the symptoms I wanted to mention and questions I didn't want to forget. Once I was in the room, I'd scribble whatever the doctor said that sounded important. Sometimes I couldn't keep up. Sometimes Scott wrote instead.

In the beginning, I brought him to almost everything. I highly recommend bringing your person—not just for moral support, but because your brain, especially if it's doing trauma, chemo, or both, is a terrible stenographer. Having someone else take notes let me be present, ask follow-ups, and occasionally remember to breathe.

That notebook became a kind of external hard drive. When I couldn't remember exactly when a side effect started, I flipped back and found it. When one doctor asked what another had called something, I could look. It made me feel less like a defendant on the witness stand and more like someone presenting evidence.

But the longer treatment went on, the less "enough" it was.

As the plan got more complex—overlapping therapies, overlapping specialists, overlapping side effects—the notebook started to show its limits. Tear-blurred ink. Half-finished questions. Margins filled with "ask about this" and arrows pointing to nowhere. I was still catching pieces of the story, but it was starting to feel like one of those conspiracy boards with red string and no legend.

I needed something I could sort. Search. Copy. Paste.

Digital Shift: Enter the Spreadsheet

The spreadsheet was born out of desperation with a side of "I cannot do this from memory anymore."

More clinics started sending intake forms online: "Please summarize your entire medical history in one paragraph or less. Don't forget your ten-digit insurance ID, every past surgery, and the exact month and year of your last abnormal scan. Also, how's your pain on a scale of 1–10?"

Meanwhile, my brain was buffering like bad Wi-Fi.

I still loved my notebook. It lived in my purse, thick with appointments and questions and half-legible scribbles. But every time I needed to find one specific detail—my Ki-67 percentage, the exact name of the drug that gave me hives, that scan where "something lit up"—I'd be flipping pages like a raccoon in a recycling bin.

So I opened a Google Sheet.

One tab became two. Two became five. Then came color-coding and filters and little drop-down menus. I added hyperlinks to patient portals. I linked to articles I didn't have the energy to reread but didn't want to lose. I started to feel less like a drowning person and more like a slightly exhausted air traffic controller.

Then something interesting happened: doctors complimented my process, and people started asking for copies. Friends. Other cancer patients. A nurse. A social worker. Turns out I wasn't the only one trying to survive cancer and also function as an unpaid care coordinator, medical historian, executive assistant, and research intern.

The spreadsheet made the whole ordeal feel 10% more manageable. Like having a map in a dark forest. Yes, you still have to walk. Yes, there are roots to trip on. But at least now you know which way is north.

System Overview: Tab by Tab

You don't have to build your system like mine, but here's the framework I landed on after a lot of trial and error (and swearing). You can do this in Excel, Google Sheets, Notion, or an app that doesn't involve grids at all. The point is not perfection; it's having a place where your story lives that isn't a stack of crumpled papers and half-remembered phone calls.

Here's how I structured mine:

Tab 1: Care Team Contacts
A directory of every provider: name, specialty, clinic, phone, address, portal URL, and any relevant notes ("only available Tuesdays," "actually listens," "bring questions in writing"). When I forget which plastic surgeon did which surgery (it's complicated), I look here instead of playing voicemail roulette.

Tab 2: Diagnosis Summary
The high-level facts I get asked about constantly:

- Date of original diagnosis
- Type and grade of cancer
- Hormone receptor status, HER2, Ki-67%
- Tumor sizes
- Key scan results
- Recurrence details

Not the long, emotional story—just the quick-download version for any new provider who needs to catch up fast. I treat it as my "press kit."

Tab 3: Current Treatment Protocol
What's going on right now:

- Meds and infusions (dosages, frequencies, route)
- Start date, projected end date
- Why I'm on it ("adjuvant chemo," "bone strength," "targeted therapy")
- Allergies and reactions in bold

Result: when someone asks, "What medications are you currently taking?" the answer is no longer "Uhhh…" followed by interpretive dance.

Tab 4: Proposed Treatment Timeline

A month-by-month view of what's ahead: chemo rounds, surgeries, scans, infusions, follow-ups. I color-coded by type (surgery, imaging, infusions, "fun thing that is not medical"). This tab gave me a way to see:

- Where things overlapped
- When I might get a break
- Why I was exhausted, beyond "because... all of this"

Tab 5: Medical History (Annual Overview)

A log of every significant appointment, scan, test, and major side effect, organized by year. I don't enter every CBC or CMP result—that's what portals are for—but I do note abnormal findings, new diagnoses, major medication changes, and hospital stays. When a doctor asks, "Have you ever had an abnormal CA 15-3?" I don't have to guess. I can search.

Tab 6: Past Treatments

Everything completed, archived but accessible:

- Which chemo agents and regimens I've had
- Surgeries (with dates and outcomes)
- Radiation fields and number of sessions
- Reactions and complications
- Whether I'd ever, ever do that again

Tab 7: Additional Medical History

All the non-cancer things that still matter: past surgeries (knee, appendix, hysterectomy), chronic conditions, allergies, relevant family history. Every new specialist wants this, and I prefer copy-paste to performing "This Is Your Medical Life" from memory.

Tab 8: Diet and Triggers (Optional)
This one is choose-your-own-adventure. Mine includes: gluten-free notes, foods that leave me wrecked, things that help (hydration, gentle movement, certain snacks).

What I Wish I'd Known Before I Started

Short version: I wish I'd started sooner.

Longer version: I had no idea how much information I'd be expected to retain, repeat, and produce on demand while also navigating grief, fear, fatigue, and whatever chemo was doing to my brain cells.

I waited until things were already tangled. Until I was flipping through my notebook in exam rooms, trying to remember what I took every morning. Until I turned to Scott and asked, "How do you spell the name of that drug I'm swallowing twice a day?" Until I sat in front of an intake form, staring at the words *last PET scan date* like they were written in a language I used to speak.

That blankness made me feel stupid. Irresponsible. Like I wasn't paying attention to my own life.

But here's the truth: this is not a personal failure. It's a system failure.

No one is meant to juggle this many moving pieces without help—and yet, that's exactly what most patients are asked to do.

If you're just starting out, or even if you're years in, here's what I wish someone had told me:

- **Start tracking early.** Before you think it's "serious enough." Before you're sure you'll remember. You won't always remember. Your future self will be so grateful you gave them a head start.
- **Don't rely on memory.** Not if you're dealing with chemo brain, trauma brain, general life exhaustion, or all of the above. Write it down. Type it out. Save it somewhere searchable and backed up.
- **You're allowed to create structure in chaos.** You don't need to be Type A or tech-savvy. You can be inconsistent and overwhelmed and still benefit. Half-finished notes are still more useful than no notes.
- **You are your strongest advocate, but you don't have to be your only one.** Systems help you invite others in: partners, friends, social workers, providers. When the fog rolls in, you'll have something to lean on besides your own exhausted brain.

The spreadsheet didn't make me invincible. It did something discerning: it helped me stop spiraling. It gave me a sense of grounding. It reminded me that struggling to remember wasn't a moral failure—it was evidence that this is simply a lot to live through.

Not All Heroes Use Google Sheets

Not everyone wants to build a tiny digital empire of tabs and conditional formatting. That's okay. I have a friend who lives by her paper calendar. She writes in doctor's appointments, kids' events, and "Bitches' Brunch" with equal commitment, and it works. Scott uses Google Keep for everything. My physical therapist records voice notes to herself and later tries to decode what "ask about shoulder weird" meant.

All valid. Here are a few patient archetypes I've met along the way (sometimes in the mirror):

- **The Color-Coder:** Lives for aesthetics. Owns more highlighters than medications. Their symptom tracker is a work of art. If they could color-code their emotions, they would.
- **The Outsourcer:** Spreadsheet? Absolutely not. That's what their sister/friend/spouse is for. Delegation is their superpower.
- **The Memory Gambler:** "It's all up here," they say, tapping their forehead—then immediately forget a Zometa infusion and show up a week late, Starbucks in hand.
- **The Journalist:** Logs everything: mood, bowel movements, dreams, lunar cycles. Possibly the stock market. Will absolutely be the one to discover a never-before-seen pattern in their own data.
- **The Post-It Prophet:** Their system is adhesive-based. Bathroom mirror, fridge, laptop, car dashboard. Reminders everywhere, like a breadcrumb trail through anarchy.

You don't have to become a Spreadsheet Person to benefit from having a system. If you're app-curious, here are a few tools patients swear by (no coding required):

- **MyChart (or your hospital's portal):** Lab results, visit summaries, meds, messages. Goldmine of data, willy-nilly interface. Expect frequent password rage.

- **CareClinic:** Symptom and medication tracking, pain, mood, routines. Clear visuals, not too fussy.
- **Bearable:** Great for chronic illness. Customizable trackers for symptoms, habits, triggers, and patterns.
- **Google Keep / Notes app:** For the minimalist. Quick, searchable, always in your purse (or pocket). Excellent for 3 a.m. "Don't forget to ask about that purple rash" thoughts.
- **Notion:** For the Type A++. Build dashboards, link pages, embed files, create the Beyoncé of illness trackers. May cause organizational euphoria... and the urge to over-design.

Try a few. Abandon what you hate. Keep what helps. The "best" system is not the fanciest one; it's the one you'll actually use on a bad day.

Diagnoses didn't come with a manual—just a branded accordion folder (in pink) and a stack of appointment cards. What I got was a whirlwind of acronyms, phone calls, and intake forms that all assumed I had immediate, flawless recall.

So I built my own manual.

Not because I wanted another project, but because being sick didn't mean I stopped being responsible. Because the system wasn't built for my brain, I built something that was.

Tracking my care gave me back something cancer and the healthcare maze both tried to steal: a sense of agency. It let me show up prepared. It let me catch things providers missed. It let me speak "doctor" when I needed to—and "human" when I didn't.

A system might create just enough room for you to rest. To cry. To laugh. To be something other than overwhelmed for a minute.

Use what helps. Toss what doesn't. Color-code if it brings you satisfaction. Dictate notes to your dog if that gets the words out. Build a dashboard or keep scribbling in the battered notebook.

The method doesn't matter. What matters is that you have a way to hold your story in your hands—literally or digitally—so you don't have to keep carrying all of it in your head.

And maybe, just maybe, you'll hand your version of that survival map to someone else one day and say, "Here. This helped me. Start wherever you are."

To the Body That Strayed–Er, Stayed

High Altitude, Oxygen Debt, and the Long Climb

Whenever I stand on the summit of a 14er, I feel two things at once: small and absurdly proud.

The mountain doesn't care that I trained. The wind doesn't care that my quads are shaking. There's no tremor of recognition—just altitude, sky, and the realization that my soft, breakable body hauled itself up one deliberate step at a time.

Cancer felt like that.

Not heroic. Not elegant. Definitely not a battle. Just a long climb through thinning air and uneven trail. One painful step, then the next, and the next.

And as I kept moving—carved, burned, poisoned, rearranged—I kept asking the same question: How is my body still doing this?

This is a trail report from high altitude. A map of switchbacks, false summits, washed-out sections, and the moments when the view stole my breath.

Because the body may stray from every familiar path—but mine stayed. And kept climbing.

Oxygen Debt: Trust

The first injury isn't a scar. It's trust.

Before cancer, my body was imperfect but legible. If something hurt, there was a reason. If I rested, it improved. If I trained, I got stronger. Cause and effect. Basic math.

Cancer broke that contract.

After that, my body didn't just hurt—it became an unreliable narrator. It could whisper "fine" while building a bonfire in the background. It could deliver good news with a caveat. It could be unrecognizable and still mine.

That's the betrayal: not the pain, not even the losses—the uncertainty. The sense that the trail itself might reroute overnight and I'm the last one to get the update.

Oxygen debt is what happens when you keep going—after your body has already spent what it has. You can still function, technically—but you're borrowing. I can't remember the last time I had a surplus of the good stuff: white blood cells, iron, hydration, energy. Every choice comes with a cost. Every cost turns into debt. The bill always shows up later.

Oxygen Debt: Signs You're Up Here

Before we zoom in, here are a few trail markers—because pretending this stuff doesn't matter does a disservice to the people living it.

Itching is the first mystery. It arrives under your skin like a rumor—a deep, unreachable itch somewhere between nerve and scar, maybe in the muscle, maybe in the soul.

Then come the other markers: Nerves firing electric zaps like a glitchy pinball machine. Fatigue pouring into your limbs like wet cement. Taste buds turning mutinous—metal, cardboard, betrayal. Vaginal dryness so intense it felt like my snatch was cracking like scorched earth.

None of this is neat. None of it follows instructions. Your body becomes unfamiliar terrain—washed out and hastily rerouted—and still you're asked to trust it.

So I'm mapping it.

If you're reading this while looking up "why does my vag feel like fire," I promise you: you're not losing it. You're just at high altitude in a body doing more work than anyone can see.

Oxygen Debt: Skin, Stitching, and the Negotiation of "Done"

I imagined surgery as a single event. Cut, create, close. Done. Like a convenience store transaction.

But the body negotiates. It resists. It reshapes. It argues with you in a language you don't speak yet.

The drains alone were their own domestic engineering project—bulbs swinging under my shirt, tubes snaking out of my sides like I'd been jury-rigged for survival.

Reconstruction wasn't a solution. It was a fork in the trail with fine print. I chose a direct-to-implant, nipple-sparing mastectomy. I was terrified of waking up flat—afraid that losing everything at once might make me disappear when I looked in the mirror.

Six months later came fat grafting. Less "body sculpting," more relocation. My thighs looked like a peach forgotten and then discovered at the bottom of a daypack.

And still—under the bruising, the swelling, the stitches—my body kept doing its work. Re-routing blood flow. Reabsorbing fluid. Stitching tissue back together like it had done this a thousand times before.

Then the mirror. Some days I avoided it entirely. Other days I stood there like I was greeting old friends I wasn't sure I recognized. This fold means healing. That shadow means swelling.

I told myself I wasn't looking for beauty. Let's be honest—I was.

And yet what kept startling me wasn't imperfection. It was adaptation.

Oxygen Debt: The Body on Meds (and Other Creative Sabotage)

Oral chemo sounds deceptively simple—no IV, no infusion room, no bell. Just a bitter tab you pop each morning.

Then your mouth revolts. Metallic tang. Velcro-textured food. Mouth sores that make toast feel weaponized.

Chemo brain wasn't confusion. It was delay. A buffering mind. Rereading texts. Forgetting mid-sentence. Staring at the espresso machine like it required a PhD.

Immunotherapy brought its own grab bag: chills in July, rashes like abstract art, fevers without warnings.

There's a particular kind of rage in taking something meant to keep you alive and discovering your body has opinions about it. Not poetic opinions. Bureaucratic ones. Denied. Not today. Try again.

This is oxygen debt too: the labor of metabolizing, filtering, compensating—your body doing triage while you're out here pretending you're fine because you answered an email.

Oxygen Debt: Hormones and the Coup

Medical menopause arrived without warning or ceremony.

"Chemo will likely induce menopause," my oncologist said casually, as if I might pencil it in between nausea and fatigue.

Hot flashes didn't walk in politely—they staged a coup. I fantasized about turning my refrigerator into a sleeping pod. I fought the urge to make snow angels in December wearing nothing but regret.

And the crying. Sweet baby Jesus, the crying.

Not sadness. Not depression. Just… overflow. Like my whole nervous system had sprung a leak.

Effexor helped. Sleep returned in cautious increments. Four uninterrupted hours felt like winning an Oscar.

Hand moisturizer became a reminder to also moisturize the vag. My Amazon recommendations got weird quickly.

Through all this disarray, my body wasn't failing. It was recalibrating after having its hormones yanked out like faulty wiring—bending, cracking, under duress.

Unrecognizable. Still mine.

Oxygen Debt: Rerouting Intimacy

I remember the first time Scott touched my nipples after surgery. His fingers moved gently. I felt pressure, but no pleasure. After a few seconds, I looked down to check: was he still touching me?

That's how strange it gets—having to visually confirm intimacy because the nerves have stopped forwarding the mail.

Sex became a strategy game. Okay to touch here, not there; this angle safe, that one a landmine. We used pillows like emotional bubble wrap—propping, adjusting, protecting skin and spirit. It wasn't exactly romantic.

But it was real.

We stayed playful. We laughed at the wrong turns. We celebrated the wins when things aligned just right. Awkward tenderness.

Intimacy became less about performance and more about willingness: to try again—just differently. The desire didn't disappear. It shapeshifted. Became gentler, slower, rooted in safety.

Some nights intimacy was a shoulder rub. Or folding laundry together—Scott doing most of it, me managing the socks with my T-rex arms.

We talked—sometimes beautifully, sometimes terribly.

"I want to feel close but I'm nervous." "This feels weird; can we pause?"

Those conversations were their own kind of intimacy. Permission to fumble without shame.

Because intimacy after cancer isn't about getting your old body back. It's about learning your new one without abandoning it.

Unrecognizable. Still mine.

Oxygen Debt: Infrastructure Damage

Radiation is often advertised as "the easy one." Localized. Predictable. Nothing like chemo.

For the first couple of weeks, I believed it. I lay still while the machine circled me, humming and pivoting, and thought: Maybe this won't be so bad.

Week four whispered: absolutely not.

Radiation fatigue descends like a weighted blanket. You crash before noon. Words slip out of reach. Even the microwave's cheerful ding feels hostile.

And the skin. The beams didn't just enter; they exited. A precise field across front, side, underboob, neck, back. Burns arrived in layers: flush, sting, peeling skin that flared when air hit it. Itching like ants performing interpretive dance under the skin.

Even after the final zap, the tightness lingered. Nerve twitches sparked. Emotionally, I felt muted. Not depressed. Just blurred around the edges from being irradiated daily for six and a half weeks.

And just as the effects of radiation were fading from memory, lymphedema arrived.

A line buried in the consent form became my new reality: heaviness, tightness, puffiness. Startling. Miserable. Infrastructure damage. The lymphatic system ghosting me at the exact moment I needed it most.

My first compression sleeve was beige—shriveled golden-raisin beige. My arm looked like a wrapped bratwurst. Later I found patterned sleeves, tattoo styles for the lymph-challenged. Funny and sad and helpful all at once.

I carry a letter for the TSA explaining the sleeve, the pump, the swelling. Cue pat-downs, chemical swabs, confused stares. Every damn time.

There was a moment with my leather jacket. It wouldn't fit over my swollen arm—tearing something open inside of me. Not because of the jacket itself, but because of everything it represented: the ways my body has to work harder now, just to exist in the same world.

This is the long tail of treatment. The altitude of consequence.

Oxygen Debt: The Pump

Zipping into the pump each night is not graceful. It requires the overhead light—because this is not a "dim lamp and soft music" situation. This is hoses and Velcro and a vest that looks like tactical gear for people whose lymphatic systems decided to go off-grid.

There are three attachment points. Three. And none of them are stitched together with thread and seams like a normal garment. It's all Velcro, so you can micro-adjust the pressure at the elbow, the forearm, the fingertips—because nothing says relaxation like negotiating airflow with your own body parts.

It's a fifty-minute interval where the machine "clears" my torso and arm in a synchrony that feels both clinical and oddly intimate. Chest first. Shoulder. Upper arm. Back to shoulder. Back to chest. Then forearm to upper arm to chest. Then fingertips to forearm to upper arm to shoulder to chest, puffing and sighing the whole way—like Darth Vader took up caregiving.

When it starts, the TV volume goes up by three. Always three. A small, predictable accommodation for the wheeze next to my ear.

We start a show as it starts clearing lymph from my chest. As the episode moves forward, my body rolls subtly with the air movement. My shoulder blades readjust to the pressure and then settle into the couch back like they're finally giving in to the load.

The pump is firm but relaxing—if you consider puffing, popping, and sighing to be a kind of white noise. A mechanical lullaby. A nightly reminder: my body is doing math I can't see.

There are rules. I can't eat right before. When the constriction moves from chest to belly, discomfort arrives in record time. I have to recline the couch before I sit down. Once I'm strapped in, I can't reach the controls. The light has to be turned off before I sit down too—same reason. Set the stage, climb into the contraption, surrender.

Some nights, tired, I wiggle into the vest, arrange the hoses so I can sit back, and ready myself to watch the show—only to hear Scott ask, "Are you going to hit start?"

I laugh. Then I swear. The idea of crawling out of my nest and back in again is overwhelming.

He hops up and starts the machine so I don't have to. That's love.

When it's over, I slither out of the contraption, put it away, and reach for my reward cookie while my arm works out the final tingles.

This is oxygen debt: you can function, but you're borrowing.

Oxygen Debt: The View from Here

When I look back at the map—the surgery, the drains, the grafts, the pills, the hormone crash, the intimacy reroutes, the swelling, the sleeves, the nightly pump—it would look like a blueprint for collapse.

That's not what happened.

This body has been carved open, burned, poisoned, rearranged, dried out, numbed, and exhausted.

Still: it laughed. It parented. It worked. It loved. It had sex. It walked through TSA. It hiked. It wrote this.

On the good days, I feel small in the best way—like someone standing on the summit, turning around to look at the route they just came up.

Small, and ferociously proud.

This isn't the body I thought I'd live in. It's the one that stayed. It is a wonder. And I'm still on the trail, moving one uneven, astonishing step at a time.

PART IV

Life, Reimagined

I Wrote This So I Wouldn't Forget

There are days I feel awe at what this body has survived. There are days I forget it.

This chapter is for the latter. (Bookmark this. Screenshot it. Tear it out. I won't mind.)

First: Rest. Then Anything Else.

You don't need to earn rest by being productive first. There isn't a cosmic scoreboard handing out extra points for showing up to life while exhausted.

Some days, survival is the task. If your body says nope, listen. Curl up. Take a nap. Close the laptop. Rest isn't quitting. Rest is how you keep going.

And yes, you might feel guilty for lying down. That's okay. Lie down anyway. Let the guilt sit in the corner and mutter to itself while you heal.

You also don't have to be anyone's silver lining. When you hear "you're so strong" or "you've got this," it's meant to help. Sometimes it does. Sometimes it lands like one more job you didn't apply for.

You don't have to be anyone's story of resilience.

You don't have to be grateful on demand.

You don't have to post your "Big Lesson" for public consumption.

You're allowed to just... be.

Angry. Scared. Sarcastic. Bored. Relieved. Over it.

Human.

And if you're used to doing it all, I get it. Cancer doesn't care. You will need help—logistical, emotional, physical, existential. You might not know what kind. Say yes anyway.

Say yes to dinner—especially if it's cheesy baked potatoes bland enough to pass over your tongue.

Say yes to company—even if you don't talk.

Say yes to the ride—even if you could technically drive yourself.

You don't have to carry all of this alone. You never did. You just forgot.

Second: Your Body Is Not Your Enemy. It's Your Home Base.

I know—sometimes it feels like your body ambushed you. Like it tricked you. Like it failed the one basic assignment of not getting cancer. That's real.

But here's the thing: your body didn't set out to ruin you. It's been doing its best to keep you here.

Even when it hurts. Even when it's scarred. Even when it feels alien.

Still yours.

It's still your body. And you don't have to love it to live in it. You can be pissed and still show up for it. That, too, is a form of healing.

It may not be the body you expected, but it's the one that stayed.

Grief and gratitude can live side by side. You can hate this and still find beauty in it. You can be thankful and furious. You can be cursing into your heating pad while the light hits your dog's face just right and your heart does that stupid, tender thing.

Contradiction has tentacles. Let it.

You might wake up numb, cry at a car ad, rage-clean your bathroom, then go absolutely deadpan while getting news that should've rattled you.

There's no right sequence. This isn't a feel-good rom-com. It's churn, not closure.

You are not required to be positive. You are not required to be okay.

You're allowed to feel like shit.

You're also allowed to laugh in chemo.

You're allowed to want both space and company.

It counts.

Feel it all. Then feel something else. That's how this works.

Third: You Deserve Answers. You Deserve Clarity. You Deserve Care Without Performing

You don't need a medical degree to deserve answers. You don't have to be polite when your survival is on the line.

Ask the question.

Ask it again.

Ask until the answer makes sense to you, not just to the person in the white coat who says it six times a day.

Ask about side effects. Ask about timelines. Ask about sex. Ask what the hell a port is and why it sounds like it belongs in a sci-fi movie.

Bring someone with you to take notes. Or record the appointment. Or mutter to yourself on the drive home while you try to remember what lymph nodes even are.

Clarity is a requirement, not a luxury.

You are not difficult. You're a patient. And you're allowed to take up space.

And please hear this one clearly: you didn't cause this.

After I was diagnosed, I became a detective. Or maybe a prosecutor. I scoured the internet for every known breast cancer risk factor and cross-examined my life like it was a crime scene.

Did I drink too much? Was it the stress I wore like a second skin? The hormonal birth control? The deodorant? The frozen pizza? The bad breakups?

I wanted a reason. A cause. A breadcrumb trail that would lead to why. But the truth? I'll never know. And neither will you.

You didn't cause this. Your thoughts didn't cause this. Your stress didn't cause this. Your personality didn't cause this.

Cancer is not a punishment. It's not karmic. It's not proof you failed at wellness. It's something that happened to you—not because of you.

You deserve compassion, not blame. Especially from yourself.

Be gentle with the you who kept going anyway. Survival is still survival, even when it doesn't look impressive.

Last, People and Systems Will Surprise You. Plan Accordingly.

Some people will step up in ways you never expected. They'll drop off flowers, send the perfect text, or say nothing at all and somehow still manage to say everything.

Others will step back so fast they leave a cartoon dust cloud. Or offer up gems like "everything happens for a reason," or "my mom's cancer just metastasized to her lungs."

You'll wonder what the hell just happened. Then you'll learn to stop expecting people to be good at this.

Let them be human. Then decide what kind of human you want near you.

Boundaries are not just allowed—they're vital. This is not the time to people-please your way into emotional collapse.

Also, cancer is administrative. Appointments. Labs. Side effects. Bills. Follow-ups. Authorizations. Insurance reps who say "ma'am" like it's a threat.

You might need a spreadsheet. A binder. A designated drawer full of prescription bottles and broken pens. You might become someone who highlights things.

It's annoying. It's dehumanizing. It helps.

You don't need to do it perfectly, just well enough to stay in the loop of your own care.

If you can delegate any part of it, do. You shouldn't have to manage this all alone—but the system will let you. And it will call that empowerment.

Hope, With a Side of Realism

There's life after diagnosis. Sometimes it looks like slow mornings, nerve pain, and eating soup in your bathrobe because everything else tastes like metal.

This isn't redemption or epiphany. There's no transcendent glow.

But there will be ordinary joy.

Belly laughs. Clean scans. A moment in the sun where you realize, Oh. I'm still here.

You can be hopeful without being delusional. You can be realistic without giving up.

Let that be enough.

One More Thing

You don't have to be brave today.

You don't have to be brave tomorrow.

You don't have to be brave at all.

You just have to be here.

You can fall apart in the shower and pull yourself together in the parking lot. You can cry because the cookies are gone, or because someone said the exact right thing in a tone that made you want to disappear.

You're still here. In a changed body. In a life that might not look anything like what you pictured ten years ago.

You don't owe anyone a comeback.

Survival doesn't mean you're done. It means you're in it. Still becoming. Still learning to live with the noise, the scars, the beauty, the boredom, the ache, the absurdity of it all.

I wrote this so I wouldn't forget: Healing isn't linear. Anger can be sacred. Joy is still possible, even if you have to squint.

Softness is a strength. Being alive—really alive—doesn't require a smile or a slogan.

Breathe.

If you're tired of being brave, let that be okay. Rest here. Come back to this when you need it. You don't have to be ready. You just have to be.

I wrote this so I wouldn't forget. And if you forget too—borrow my words until yours come back.

I'm here. On the page. On the hard days.

Tools for the Chronic Unknown

Cancer has an "after," but it's not the credits rolling. It's not the montage where you go back to work with a new lease on life and great hair.

It's scans. Pains. Reminders for labs, PT, and Zometa infusions. It's watching the calendar, the clock, your own body. It's living in that blurry stretch of maybe.

This isn't post-cancer freedom—it's post-treatment vigilance.

The long middle: not in crisis anymore, but not fine either.

You might be NED (no evidence of disease), which technically means remission—but it can feel less like relief and more like purgatory. Like waiting. Like listening for a sound you can't name.

Your life stops being organized around treatment, but it's still shaped by it. You're back in the world, sort of—except your nervous system is pacing the perimeter like a guard dog who doesn't trust the neighborhood anymore.

This chapter is here to offer tools—small, imperfect things that make it more livable.

The Long Middle

People around you exhale and say, "I'm so glad it's over," while your nervous system is still on the night shift. Your scans are clear, but your sleep is nonexistent. Your hair might be growing back, but your faith in your body is not. There's no schedule for how long you'll feel off balance. No bell to ring every time you make it through another scan cycle without emotional upheaval in the driveway.

This is survivorship. Not the pinkwashed version—the real thing. And it takes tools. The kind that help you stay in your body without abandoning yourself every time it twitches.

Tool 1: Vigilance vs. Hypervigilance

After cancer, you're told to stay vigilant: report new symptoms, be your own advocate, keep an eye on things.

But how do you do that without spiraling?

Every sensation becomes suspect.

Headache? Brain mets.

Hip pain? Bone mets.

Fatigue? Recurrence. Again.

Vigilance keeps you safe. Hypervigilance keeps you trapped. The line between the two is razor-thin and constantly moving.

Recently, I broke out in hives—bad ones. I've had chronic urticaria since chemo, but this was different: more hives, larger, longer-lasting, arriving without a clear trigger. So I did what any rational, formerly cancerous human with Wi-Fi and dread would do: I Googled.

Not "hives + cancer."

"Bed bugs."

We were staying in a motel. My husband had zero bites. I was covered. I scrolled through infestation photos, learned way too much about mattress seams, and mentally drafted a complaint to the front desk—all while staring at hives that looked nothing like bug bites.

Bed bugs were horrifying. But at least they weren't systemic. At least they didn't show up on a scan.

That's what hypervigilance can look like. You'd rather believe you're infested with blood-sucking insects than consider that your immune system is misfiring again.

If you're hypervigilant, it doesn't mean you're delusional or broken. It means your body tried to kill you or hosted something that did, and your nervous system is still on the night shift.

The tool here isn't "calm down." It's stay with yourself:

- Name what you're afraid of—and what else it might be.
- Have one or two trusted people you can reality-check with.
- Set a hard rule for escalation. Don't decide in the panic of the moment. Decide now.

My rule was the Trifecta: New. Lasting. Worsening. If a symptom hits all three, the debate is over.

The tool is learning how to stay awake without burning yourself alive.

Tool 2: Rituals That Regulate

There's no onboarding process for your new nervous system. No orientation video titled So You've Survived—Now What?

You improvise.

Some of my rituals are tiny:

- I play the same playlist on the way to PET scans and while the radioactive serum settles in.
- I drink something warm before blood draws, even if it's 85 degrees out.
- I bring my Death Cab for Cutie chemo hoodie to appointments—not because it's lucky, but because it zips easily and shields me from institutional air-conditioning.

These little signals say to my body: We're here. You're not alone. We can get through this hour.

Other rituals are bigger:

- Five minutes of breathwork on the couch for before I open the first portal message after a scan.
- A walk in the sun when my brain wants to scroll.
- Stretching before bed because my shoulders forget what "down" feels like.

Call it self-care. Call it "things I do so I don't lose my shit at Walgreens." Either way, it counts.

Micro-tool (portal dread): don't read results alone, in the dark, at 11:47 p.m. Daylight if you can. A person if you can. At minimum: two slow breaths before you click.

Tool 3: Stewardship (Nourish, Move, Rest)

After cancer, food, movement, and rest stop being items on the wellness checklist and start feeling more like negotiations.

I used to think in terms of "getting it right"—the right diet, the right workout, the right sleep routine. Cancer blew that up.

Now the question is simpler: Does this help me stay in my body today?

Nourish. Whole foods aren't a flex; they're a resource. My body has been through chemical warfare and early-onset menopause. Protein helps me protect my bones. Colorful, minimally processed foods support my energy and inflammation. Hydration is how I put the fire out. This isn't about restriction. It's about restoration: eating like someone who wants to stick around.

Move. Movement used to mean miles and elevation. Now it means connection. Some days it's a walk around the block or dancing in the kitchen for one song. Other days it's a calculated risk: training for a hard hike, knowing I might pay for it later but choosing the challenge anyway. It's less "prove what your body can do" and more "remember you have a body at all."

Rest. Post-cancer fatigue is not regular tired; it's a full-system shutdown. I've stopped treating rest as a reward and started treating it as a treatment. If I can't sleep, I still lie down. I let my body exist without performing. There's nothing lazy about this. It's choosing not to override the check-engine light.

You don't have to do any of this perfectly. Stewardship isn't about control. It's about care.

Tool 4: Connection, on Your Terms (and Permission to Disappear)

After treatment, people assume you're ready to "come back." What they don't see is how foreign everything feels now—including you.

Connection gets weird. You might crave people and feel overstimulated by them at the same time. You might miss your old life and feel allergic to small talk and "You're better now, right?" cheerfulness.

Here's the tool: you set the terms.

- You're allowed to say no to plans that drain you, even if you "look fine."
- You're allowed to mute group texts and answer when you have the bandwidth.
- You're allowed to grieve the relationships that didn't survive your cancer, without forcing yourself to rebuild them.

Some connections deepen: the friend who can have a raw, honest conversation; the fellow survivor who gets it without explanation; the stranger on a message board at 2 a.m.

Sometimes connection looks like letting someone watch you fall apart and… and then exist.

And when you don't have that? Solitude can be sacred too. You're not meant to do this alone—but you're allowed to be alone while you figure out how to do this.

Boundaries are a tool.

Tool 5: Conscious Coping

My relationship with alcohol didn't end in a dramatic rock-bottom story. It just…shifted.

Chemo made everything with a "bite" taste like battery acid. By the time my mouth recovered, I'd already gotten used to sober living. Then recurrence showed up—triple negative, aggressive. I wasn't doing chemo to keep drinking; I was doing chemo to stay alive. So alcohol became rare: a birthday mezcal, a cocktail on vacation, not a nightly cope.

I tried cannabis edibles. Sometimes they helped with sleep and pain. Sometimes they turned the volume up on my anxiety and left me feeling like a squirrel having an existential crisis. Eventually I realized I wasn't regulating; I was just rearranging deck chairs.

The tool here is know your why:

- Why am I reaching for this right now?
- Does it actually help me regulate, or does it just blur the edges?
- How do I feel the day after—in my body and in my brain?

I don't believe in blanket rules for everyone. I believe in informed choices, made with your actual body and actual life in mind. Not clean. Conscious.

Tool 6: Hope, With Boundaries

There's a version of hope that says, "Everything will be okay." And there's a version that says, "I don't know what's coming, but I trust myself to face it."

I live in the second one now. It took a shit ton of therapy to get here.

For a long time, every time I looked forward to something—school, a honeymoon, a trip—cancer canceled it. Especially when recurrence showed up like a terrible encore. It felt dangerous to hope for anything.

Hope, these days, looks tender:

- Planning epic hikes months ahead while a small part of me still whispers: what if.

- Letting myself imagine future vacations, a new career, my kids' milestones.
- Staying in relationship with my body even when it confuses or scares me.

Hope needs boundaries too. You can be hopeful and still say no. Grateful and still tired. Believe in your healing and still have a spreadsheet, a therapist, and a backup plan.

There's no finish line here. Just the rhythm of living in the unknown, one choice at a time.

You're not failing if you're still figuring it out. You're not lost—you're living through it.

This is survivorship: raw, infuriating, extraordinary.

Agency in the Aftermath

Survivorship comes with a strange promise: one day, things will settle.

You'll get far enough from treatment that your body remembers how to function, your brain stops the endless scanning for danger, and your calendar becomes something other than a medical scavenger hunt.

Yet survivorship doesn't settle. It mutates.

You learn to live with the chronic unknown—the unglamorous stretch where life looks ordinary from the outside and your nervous system keeps one eye on the door. Where you're "doing great, all things considered," but one click, one pill, one phone call can send you spinning.

It's also about something survivorship rarely gets credit for: Agency.

Agency.

The authority to decide what happens to your body, even if others raise their eyebrows or hope you'll choose differently.

I need to share two stories—one about returning fear, and one about treatment becoming the threat.

Together, they're the ground I've been walking.

The Haunting of Scanxiety

Once scanxiety learns your address, it forwards all your mail.

Every PET, every blood draw, every imaging report sits like a paperweight on your week. Does scanxiety get easier with time, like exposure therapy? It doesn't. You just learn to function through it—make jokes, attend work, forget for half an hour that your future might pivot on a radiologist's summary.

After recurrence, vigilance started feeling like instinct.

When new results drop into the chart, you don't necessarily panic. You brace. You read. You research. Recognition arrives before emotion—oh, this again—because your body already has the muscle memory of the dance.

As the summer of my second year NED unfolded, I was deep in graduate school and gratefully immersed in regular life. On a Sunday afternoon, my portal pinged during family time in the living room. I'd been calm going into the scan and was fine waiting for results.

Hope whispered: Please, let it be nothing.

Instead: spiculated. Increased uptake. Possible recurrence.

Fuck.

My face stayed put. I found Scott in the kitchen and whispered the results didn't look great. Then I did what survivors do—I logged into our weekly family Discord call, laughed in the right places, and held my gaze steady.

I didn't just carry my fear; I carried theirs.

My son was starting a new job in the morning—I told him the results hadn't posted yet. My stepdaughter had interviews the next day, so I stayed neutral.

It wasn't deceit. It was love metabolized into stoicism.

After the call, I sat with the report. Then I read about the report—SUV values, inflammatory artifacts, case studies. I wasn't spiraling; I was gathering data, building mental models, looking for the line between "monitor" and "mobilize."

Beneath the analysis was a reticent truth: How is this my normal? How is "possible recurrence" now just Sunday business?

In the end, my oncologist's call delivered the verdict: likely inflammatory changes within the radiation field. My breast surgeon concurred. We'd watch, not panic. The headline shifted from "possible recurrence" to "probably fine, but let's keep an eye on it."

My body didn't get that memo right away. The adrenaline, the bracing, the long night of what-ifs—those stayed.

With a scan, the threat was what might be there. With a blackout, the threat was what was supposed to keep it away.

When the Treatment Becomes the Threat

Six days after reaching the full dose of abemaciclib, I felt... tolerable. For the first time, that seemed possible. I'd just been in Denver the day before telling my oncologist that the adjustment was rough—headaches, nausea, the internal GI "squirting juice" festival, constipation—but manageable.

The next day it happened. I felt mildly uneasy but otherwise normal. A scheduler called to arrange my next PET. During the call, a wave hit me—fast and hot. Gut to face. Sweating. A flush of impending diarrhea. I rushed through the instructions—no exercise the day before, no food the day of, water only—and hurried toward the bathroom.

I don't remember making it inside.

I remember waking up on the floor. Horizontal. Disoriented. Facing the bottom of the bathroom door, staring through that tiny crack where the mud room was just barely visible.

My brain was slow to boot. A few long seconds passed before I realized: I'm lying down. Something hurt. Everything felt wrong.

As I lifted my face, I saw the blood. Bright, vivid, pooled under me.

My stomach lurched with urgency—instinct insisting I get to the toilet—but nothing happened. Instead, trembling, I pulled myself upright enough to see the mirror.

Blood smeared across my chin, dripping onto my fingers, streaked through my hair. My mouth a red slash. I slumped back down beside the small crimson pool and yelled for Scott.

He opened the door to find me slouched on the tile, bleeding and dazed. I can't imagine the spike of fear he must have felt seeing me like that. He grabbed a towel, pressed it to my mouth, and helped me out of the fog while I tried to explain I had blacked out.

Urgent care stitched my lip—five sutures. They asked what medication I was on, and my brain refused to supply the information. Fortunately, I had a Google Keep file titled "Cancer: Important Shit," and handed my phone over while I sat there shaking.

Next came the emergency dentist. X-rays showed a fractured bone above my front teeth—two teeth rammed out of their sockets, one slightly shifted, one more loosened. With intense concentration and equally intense force, he pushed the teeth back into position and splinted the whole top row with wire. I'd be returning weekly, hoping the nerves weren't completely severed and recovery was possible.

An oncology nurse sent us to the ED for a CT scan of my brain. More tests. More bloodwork. A concussion, but no dehydration. No broken arm. A strange shadow on my chest X-ray that "might need follow-up." Orthostatic testing? Perfect. In the end, no one could explain what happened.

Eleven hours later, I returned home.

The next few days were a haze of concussion recovery—slow, disjointed, surreal. I was exhausted, sore, and newly aware that my body could simply abandon me without warning.

Underneath the shock, I felt something closer to betrayal: I had agreed to suffer side effects to stay alive. I had not agreed to this.

Agency doesn't usually show up in the middle of an emergency. It sneaks in after, when the dust settles and you're left with a question that won't leave.

For me it was this: Is this treatment hurting me more than protecting me?

Risk Reduction for People With Faces

There's a myth in the cancer world that the people who "really want to live" do everything. Every pill. Every infusion. Every brutal tradeoff. Every percentage point of risk reduction.

But sometimes the bravest choice is stepping back. Not from hope. Not from care. But from harm.

My oncologist brings expertise. I bring my bones, my face, my concussion, my family, my body, my limits, my actual life. We meet in the middle.

The decision to stop targeted therapy sounds simple: I decided to stop. The truth was hardly clear: spreadsheets and evidence and the kind of conversations you don't want to be having at forty-nine.

On paper, targeted therapy offered a small additional survival benefit. In reality, it ruined my days and introduced my skull to the floor.

I went to the numbers.

I dug into peer-reviewed studies and tried to overlay them on my very non-textbook case. Mixed ER+/triple-negative biology. Early recurrence. Oophorectomy. Anastrozole. NED for more than two years. I did the statistics, eyeballed the confidence intervals, tried to tease out what any of it actually meant for me.

Stripped of pharma gloss, the math said this: staying on a CDK4/6 inhibitor might lower my recurrence risk by a sliver—a few percentage points—on top of the protections I already had from surgery and endocrine therapy. Not zero. Not huge. A nudge.

The numbers were sobering but also clarifying. They showed me the ceiling of what this drug could do for me. They also showed me the floor of what I was already doing: oophorectomy plus anastrozole, the heavy hitters of estrogen suppression, working on the part of my cancer that still listens to hormones at all.

What the math couldn't tell me was how to price my days.

How do you quantify the cost of fatigue that flattens you by three p.m., headaches that won't leave, a foggy brain that makes you feel stupid, a GI tract that dictates the shape of your day? How do you measure a drug that turns every plan into a risk assessment—*Can I hike? Can I paddle? Can I travel?*—and then literally knocks you unconscious?

On one side of the scale: a small, uncertain survival benefit. On the other: my safety, my functioning, my actual life.

My logic brain kept coming back to the same conclusion: the daily sacrifice was too great for the return. When the side effects of treatment are stripped away, I'm in very good health for someone who's had two rounds with cancer. This may be the best health I get for the rest of my life, with normal aging layered on top. Do I really want to spend two years on a drug that limits my ability to explore, contribute, create, and be a fully engaged mom, partner, and friend?

My body was drawing a boundary.

The 2 a.m. Cross-Examination

Numbers are one thing. Fear is another.

As I worked through the studies and my risk calculations, the question I finally asked myself was this: If I have a recurrence in the next three years, will I blame myself? Will I believe that my choice to stop targeted therapy caused it?

The answer came quickly: No.

First, the data are honest about their limits. Targeted therapy reduces risk over a population, but it doesn't erase it. People recur on and off the drug. There is no version of this path where I get a guarantee.

Second, we already know the single most important treatment for my situation is continuing the aromatase inhibitor—anastrozole—to keep estrogen suppressed. That, I am committed to. Eight more years, ten more years, whatever the evidence recommends. I can live with a small pill and creaky joints. I cannot live with regular blackouts and the ongoing threat of dental reconstruction.

After I did all this math—risk curves, percentages, best- and worst-case scenarios—I took it to my oncologist. I don't know what I was expecting—a list of things I hadn't considered or maybe a look of disappointment for walking away from maximum treatment. Instead, she listened. She asked clarifying questions. She looked at my calculations and, more importantly, at me. And then she said, simply:

You gave your best to these drugs. They didn't work out for you. I support your decision either way.

No shaming. No second guessing. Just a clear acknowledgment that my body and my life are part of the clinical picture.

I chose to stop.

Not taper. Not "see how it goes at a lower dose." We had already tried that; my body still felt unsafe, and there was no assurance the blackouts wouldn't come back. I drew the line.

You'd think that would be the end of it: decision made, relief achieved, move on.

Instead, I lay awake while my brain conducted a vigorous cross-examination.

Did I really try hard enough? Yes, says the logic brain. You tried until your liver was in distress and you lost consciousness and smashed your face.

Will I be disappointing anyone by not continuing? Letting people down? No, says the logic brain. Most people have no idea how you've come this far, endured this much.

Am I a quitter? No. You are an informed decision-maker, weighing risk, benefit, and the actual conditions of your life.

These are the conversations I now have with myself at two a.m.

The panic still comes in waves. Fear of making the wrong choice. Fear of future scans. Fear of the story where I stop the drug and something terrible happens anyway. It bubbles up like an underwater volcano—forceful, smoldering, utterly unconcerned with my carefully reasoned spreadsheets.

But then logic and something deeper—call it intuition, or maybe just self-respect—regain their grip. They remind me:

> You will have more energy to be the partner, mother, and friend you want to be. The conversations that happen at six p.m.—the ones you've been too exhausted to fully join—can become richer again.
>
> The daily feelings of "stupid" will ease as your brain clears. You'll have more lucidity, more creativity, more access to the parts of yourself that make life feel like yours.
>
> Your plans for the future won't orbit bathroom locations and immune suppression. You can make plans around trailheads and rivers and long drives instead.

And it's not just vibes. I've seen the research: people with a higher quality of life often live longer. Not because they meditate their tumors away, but because feeling better improves everything—movement, sleep, immunity, mood, relationships, adherence to the treatments that actually help.

The question isn't "survival benefit versus feeling better." It's "a tiny additional survival benefit versus meaningful gains in function, safety, mood, cognition, relationships, and long-term resilience."

Physical recovery means my fatigue, GI symptoms, and sleep improve; my muscles rebuild; my risk of falling drops.

Emotional and psychological recovery means less anxiety from daily side effects, fewer trauma alarms going off in my nervous system, more capacity for executive functioning, sexual health, and intimacy.

Functional recovery means I can work more reliably, parent with a fuller tank, participate in daily life without planning an evacuation route from every room.

When I lay it out this way, it's obvious: I am not abandoning treatment. I am optimizing well-being, safety, and long-term recovery. My desires are medically relevant, not a footnote.

This is what agency looks like in survivorship—not getting to choose what happened to my body, but choosing, as clearly as I can, what I am and am not willing to sacrifice next.

The Mindful Work of Choosing

If you flipped through my cancer notebook right now, you'd see the evidence of this decision in ink: not just numbers and hazard ratios, but little questions scribbled in the margins.

What is this actually buying me? What has it already cost? If my best friend were in my exact position, what would I tell her to do?

The same questions, written different ways on different days, until the answers lined up in more than one column: head, gut, heart.

Survivorship requires tools—emotional, logistical, medical. These are mine, for now. They won't show up on a scan or in an abstract, but they're what keep me honest with myself when the next decision comes.

And if you're here too—staring at a pill bottle, running your own numbers, feeling both terrified and certain—you're doing the hard work of deciding what your one life is worth.

In this long after of treatment, I don't control the risk that remains. I do control how much of my one life I'm willing to hand over to a drug that's already taken too much.

And, at least for now, I'm choosing my face, my liver, my bones, and the life I still get to live.

I am learning to trust the life I choose, even when I choose it trembling.

Radical Acceptance and the Life I Didn't Choose (But Chose Anyway)

Resistance: The Grip

When I was first diagnosed, I didn't pray. I requested my pathology reports, then I sobbed—hard, ugly, unimpressive sobbing that did not deserve a pink ribbon. Then I wiped my face and read.

Comedonecrosis. Multifocal microinvasion. Words that sounded like villains in a Marvel movie, except the plot was my chest.

I opened PubMed and started hunting. I read studies with the intensity of a hawk and the tenderness of a forklift. I highlighted terms, cross-checked statistics, clicked citations like they were trapdoors. If information could save me, I was going to out-read cancer by force of will.

This is what resistance looked like in my body: jaw clenched, shoulders braced, breath shallow—holding myself tight because I believed if I didn't, everything would fall apart.

I'm not a person of faith in the traditional sense. Science is my scaffolding: scans, data, evidence—something solid enough to grab when my insides start free-falling. In the cancer world, I watched how other people made meaning. Prayer. Divine timing. Circles of hands. Scriptures. Hope spoken aloud. My version was peer-reviewed and downloadable.

Different beliefs. Same human move: reach for a tether.

Distilled insight: Resistance isn't weakness. It's a survival strategy. It protected me when I didn't know how to soften. I see you, resistance. You once kept me alive.

And then—eventually—I got tired of proving strength through exhaustion.

The Turn: The Day I Stopped Negotiating

The moment didn't look like a spiritual awakening. It looked like me in a therapist's office, sitting on the same couch I'd sat on dozens of times, saying some version of "Are you fucking kidding me?" with a voice that had stopped expecting comfort.

My therapist listened, then said a phrase I'd never heard before: **radical acceptance.**

Two words. No glitter. No incense. No "everything happens for a reason." Just a tuning fork of language that struck something in my ribcage.

I don't remember what we were discussing—specific fear, specific frustration—but I remember the way those words stayed. They didn't explain cancer. They didn't make it mean something. They just refused to cooperate with my mental argument against reality.

I went home and did what I do: researched. But this time, not to outsmart the situation—just to understand what the phrase was asking of me.

Radical acceptance is this: **fully and completely accepting reality as it is—without denial, resistance, or judgment—even when it's painful or unfair.** It doesn't mean you like it. It doesn't mean you approve. It means you stop arguing with reality.

You can radically accept a diagnosis, a betrayal, an injustice—without forgiving, without minimizing, without calling it "meant to be."

For me, it meant this brutal simplicity: cancer was in my body. Not right, not wrong. Just true.

Distilled insight: Acceptance isn't surrender to illness. It's surrender to what is. Pain is inevitable; the second layer—the fight with reality—is optional. And I had already suffered enough.

Integration: The Afterbody, Annotated

I sat with my journal open, the morning light hitting the pages in a way that made the ink look wet. For months, I'd been trying to write my way back to the woman I was before the biopsy, before the recurrence, before the new math. But that morning, the pen felt different.

I wasn't writing a wish list anymore. I was taking a census of a new country.

Later, I looked at the scars in the mirror—the uneven line across my chest that used to make me look away. Now, I traced it. It wasn't a flaw to be corrected by a surgeon's revision. It was proof. My body was telling a story of survival, and for the first time, I didn't feel the need to edit the prose.

That afternoon, the brain fog rolled in—thick and uninvited. I had a paper due and the words wouldn't line up. The old me—the scrappy biter—would've forced it. Would've muscled through until I broke and then called it "discipline."

Instead, I practiced the radical part.

I closed the laptop. I didn't apologize to the empty room. I didn't call myself lazy or dramatic or weak. I acknowledged the truth: my energy was finite, and I was choosing to spend the rest of it on a nap.

That nap was a boundary. A vote for who I am now.

And here's where the shadows showed up. Not villains—defenders.

Envy. Resentment. Impatience. Criticism.

Envy wasn't pettiness—it was longing. It pointed to what still mattered.

Resentment wasn't cruelty. It was exhaustion with the performance of being "fine."

Impatience was life force—refusing to rot quietly in waiting rooms.

Criticism tried to perfect me before anyone else could hurt me. Protective. Misguided. Familiar.

And the lopsidedness? A reshaped version of wholeness. Not symmetrical. But mine.

Distilled insight: The parts I tried to hide still served me. They weren't stains. They were signals—bright flags pointing toward what I value, what I miss, what I won't pretend doesn't hurt. I can thank them for their honesty without handing them the nervous system.

This is what it looks like, living in the afterbody: softer in the jaw, firmer in the boundaries, and finally loyal to the truth.

Choice: The Life I Didn't Choose, Chosen Anyway

I didn't choose cancer. I didn't choose recurrence. I didn't choose the way my calendar turned medical, the way "normal" became a rumor.

But one morning, I sat at the kitchen table with my laptop open and my notes beside me—bullet points, names, facts. My phone was on speaker. I was waiting to be connected to my state representative's office.

There's a particular kind of hold music that makes you feel like you're trapped inside a corporate aquarium.

When someone finally answered, I didn't do the old thing—polite, compliant, careful not to be "too much." I didn't soften the edges so my pain could be palatable.

I spoke plainly about health disparities. About access. About the cruelty of systems that pretend illness is a personal failure. My voice didn't shake—not because I wasn't emotional, but because I was done auditioning for permission.

When I hung up, I realized something: radical acceptance hadn't made me passive. It had made me available—for my own life, for truth, for impact.

This shift wasn't only political. It was relational.

It was in the way I sat with my kids and listened to their storms without trying to be the lightning rod that absorbed it all. I stopped mistaking suffering for usefulness. I practiced being the dock—sturdy, present—letting them navigate their own water while I stayed near.

It was in the way I approached my work and my future: not as a rigid timeline I had to "get back on," but as a path that could evolve without erasing me.

When my diagnosis derailed my path in respiratory therapy, I didn't retreat to the place of safety. I took a breath, reassessed, and chose a direction rooted in purpose. I earned my BS in Lifestyle Medicine, because I believe in the daily, unglamorous work of health. And while receiving treatment in the cancer clinic, I watched social workers doing the work of presence—translating crisis into care, holding the human in the system.

A new path clarified: health social work.

I also became harder to manipulate with guilt. Easier to love with honesty. More willing to walk away from what depletes me. My energy is precious now. So is my time.

I don't tolerate cruelty disguised as tradition. But I don't meet it with rage, either. I've learned the power of calm, rational truth—the kind that holds its ground without hardening its heart.

And I notice beauty everywhere—especially in what's overlooked. The subtle shifts of light. The wild resilience of color. The exquisite details that remind me life is still offering itself, even to an altered body.

Distilled insight: Acceptance is not resignation. Acceptance is the ground you stand on when you choose your next step with eyes open. The life I didn't choose is still my life—and I get to choose how I inhabit it.

Final Vow: My Terms

I used to miss my old self—the body, the stamina, the fierce independence. She was scrappy. A biter. Underestimated. She didn't ask for help. She didn't need to. She was a model of tenacity.

Now I know better.

That old self didn't yet understand the strength it takes to soften. To be seen. To trust. To let other people love you without paying for it in exhaustion.

This version of me is still strong—just not in the way people prefer.

She doesn't audition for resilience. She doesn't make suffering look noble.

She doesn't hustle for worth. She doesn't perform "fine." She doesn't translate her pain into something easier to swallow.

She won't apologize for needing help. She won't carry other people's discomfort like it's her job. She won't confuse endurance with virtue.

She is selectively interdependent—because connection beats performance. Because love is not a transaction. Because being "low maintenance" is not a moral achievement.

Unbound. Unhidden. Fully here.

I didn't choose cancer. But I choose this life—every day—with discernment, with presence, with love. That is radical acceptance.

That is the story I am writing.

Epilogue: A Letter to the Ones Who Carried Me

There are a thousand ways to survive cancer, but not one of them is solitary. Whatever strength I had was braided with yours.

This isn't my first thank-you to you—not even close—but it may be the truest. The one written with a clearer mind, a fuller heart, and a deeper understanding of what your care actually meant.

To every person who loved on me over the past few years—this is for you.

You may not think of yourself as a caregiver. You were "just" helping. "Just" showing up in the ugly moments. "Just" doing what needed to be done.

But you made me feel human again.

You let me cry and didn't wince. You let the silence stretch. Sometimes you even cried with me. It wasn't about fixing anything. It was about staying.

You fed me—not just kindly, but smartly. You asked what I could eat. You made real food. You portioned it out in containers I didn't have to return (a saintly move). You thought about texture, temperature, smell. You thought about me.

You made it fresh. Flowers, candles, clean counters. Sunlight in the kitchen. You turned my bunker of a house into something softer.

You showed up. You drove me. Sat with me in waiting rooms. Hung out while I was under anesthesia. You didn't just drop off enchiladas—you stayed.

You knew when to laugh. You went dark with me, matching my morbid jokes beat for beat. And the Fuck Cancer socks and peppermint foot balm? A+ caregiving swag. Chemo couture at its finest.

You let me feel useful. You watered the plants with me, following my instructions like we were conducting botanical surgery. It gave me purpose.

You helped me rest without making a thing of it. You asked, "What do you need today?" And then you didn't take it personally when I changed my mind an hour later.

You made me feel seen—not just as a patient, but as myself. You brought the mastectomy pillow I didn't know I needed. You researched. Anticipated. Noticed what was missing and filled the gap.

You grieved with me. You let the pain be real. You sat in the dark with me—no headlamp, no pep talk, no rush to turn the light on.

You cared for my body when I couldn't. You stripped drains, helped me bathe, pulled shirts over my aching arms. You adjusted pillows, positioned recliners, walked with me like we were wading through molasses—slow and steady.

You spoke for me when I had no words. You made calls, filled out forms, explained things. But you still looked to me.

You checked in with your eyes. You nodded, including me in the quiet. That mattered.

You carried things I didn't always see—your fear, your exhaustion, your own heartbreak—and you still showed up anyway.

You helped me write this damn book, literally and metaphorically. Your care stitched me back together, piece by piece, day by day. You gave me back parts of myself I thought I'd lost.

Caregiving isn't glamorous. It's not sexy. But it's cherished. And exhausting. And world-shifting.

If you are reading this and you cared for me—whether by making soup, driving me to treatment, texting "I'm thinking about you," or just sitting with me in the hard spaces—please know: these words don't come close.

You didn't just make life easier. You made life possible.

I am here—creating, learning, dreaming, writing—because your fingerprints are all over my healing. I carry your care in my cells, in my nervous system, in how I now show up for others.

I can't repay you. But I can honor you—in the life you helped give back to me.

And I do.

Acknowledgments

There are people who carried pieces of this story long before I found the language for it. This book exists because I didn't have to survive any of this alone.

To Scott—my constant in the chaos and calm. You held joy, fear, absurdity, and uncertainty with me in equal measure. You gave me steadiness when my world was spinning. Thank you for showing up with devotion, curiosity, and a sense of humor that never once failed me. You made the unbearable bearable and the ordinary sublime.

To my children and stepchildren—you met this diagnosis with honesty, vulnerability, and a kind of courage that looked different in each of you. You asked hard questions. You shared dark humor with me when it was needed most. You let yourselves feel it, even when it hurt. Max, thank you for the rides to appointments, for the everyday care, and for taking on more than anyone your age should have to. To all of you—you reminded me that love grows up right along with us.

To my family and chosen family—your presence, care packages, texts, and perfectly timed humor stitched me back together. Even when we weren't in the same room, I felt you.

To my oncology team—surgeons, nurses, techs, social workers, schedulers, receptionists, and the humans who run the clinic with the precision of a NASA launch pad—thank you for saving my life in every small and enormous way. You held the clinical and the human with equal grace. You tolerated my spreadsheets and my many, many questions.

To my therapist—thank you for teaching me how trauma lives in the body and how compassion can live beside it, and for holding space where I could tell the truth without performing strength. Our work helped me move from surviving to integrating, and I carry that forward every day.

To the women and survivors who came before me and beside me—you gave me a map when I wasn't sure I had a future. Your honesty made room for my own.

To the readers who pick up this book—whether you're in the middle of treatment, living in the long after, supporting someone who is, or simply trying to understand—thank you for being here. I hope something in these pages helps you feel less alone, more seen, or more capable of asking for the care you deserve.

And to the version of me who kept writing through the scans, the setbacks, the fatigue, and the fear—you made it. I'm proud of you.

Take a Small Step Today

Learn

Choose one small thing to get curious about—your health, your healing, your boundaries, your story. Curiosity is its own power.

Attend

Show up for something that supports you—a support group, a class, a conversation, or a moment of stillness.

Volunteer

Offer what you have—an hour, a skill, a listening ear, a vote, a voice. Contribution reminds us we can create change, even in small doses.

Connect

Choose one relationship or connection to nurture today—your community, your support system, your closest circle. Healing deepens when it moves in both directions.

Empowerment rarely arrives all at once.
It grows from one small step, repeated with care.

About the Author

Jill Wilson is a two-time breast cancer survivor, a human rights advocate, and an author who prefers truth over pink ribbons. A Master of Social Work (MSW) student and board member for the United Nations Association of Boulder County, she blends lifestyle medicine principles with a fierce commitment to patient agency and health equity.

She wrote *Off My Chest* to challenge the "warrior" narrative and offer a practical, unvarnished companion for anyone navigating the chronic unknown.

Jill lives in Longmont, Colorado, with her husband, Scott, and their blended family—including a teenage daughter, a son in his twenties, and a rotating cast of grown children who ensure the house is never quiet. A believer in radical acceptance and calculated risk, she's busy reclaiming her body through adventure—most recently hiking the full 20-mile Narrows in Zion National Park and planning a 14er summit to celebrate a long-awaited NED milestone. When the world slows down, you can find her at her pottery wheel, painting, or in search of the conversations that make life make sense.

Made in the USA
Coppell, TX
01 March 2026

73011326R00146